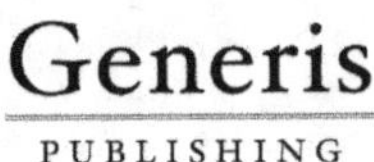

Generis
PUBLISHING

Network Neurophysiology

B.A. Lobasyuk
A.V. Zamkovaya
A.N. Stoyanov

Title: **Network Neurophysiology**

ISBN: 979-8-89248-987-4

Author: B.A. Lobasyuk, A.V. Zamkovaya,A.N. Stoyanov

Cover image: B.A. Lobasyuk

Publisher: Generis Publishing
Online orders: www.generis-publishing.com
Contact email: info@generis-publishing.com

Lobasyuk B.A., Barcewicz L.B., Zamkovaya A. V., Stoyanov O.M.

Network Neurophysiology

Odessa 2025

5

Lobasyuk B.A., Barcewicz L.B. Zamkovaya A. V., Stoyanov O.M. Network Neurophysiology, Odessa 2025.

UDC

Using multiple regression and correlation analysis methods, as well as two-dimensional correlation analysis, the relationships between the amplitudes and frequencies of EEG rhythms were studied both within a single lead and between different leads in individuals with normal development, individuals with intellectual disabilities, left-handers, and right-handers. Multiple regression equations were geometrically interpreted using polycyclic multigraphs.

As a result of the study and calculations, it was found that left-handers exhibit a greater number of multiple regression coefficients — both in calculations within a single lead between different EEG rhythms and within a single rhythm between different leads.

The study and calculations also established that in individuals with intellectual disabilities, the number of regression and two-dimensional correlation coefficients is higher than in individuals with normal development. In left-handed individuals with intellectual disabilities, the number of multiple regression coefficients was lower than in right-handed individuals with intellectual disabilities, but the number of two-dimensional correlation coefficients was higher. The observed increase in the number of correlation coefficients may indicate an elevated tone in left-handed individuals with intellectual disabilities compared to right-handed individuals with intellectual disabilities.

The highest number of regression relationships between different leads was found between the amplitudes of the alpha rhythm, with both positive and negative relationships identified. This may indicate the presence of multiple stationary generators (at least two) of the alpha rhythm, operating at close frequencies but with different phases, as well as the fact that the alpha rhythm amplitude indices used in the analysis belong to a single set of indicators. In the regression analysis of other EEG rhythms, polycyclic multigraphs were not constructed. This may suggest that the generators of other EEG rhythms are multiple.

Keywords: left-handers, right-handers, intellectual disability; multiple regression, polycyclic multigraphs.

TABLE OF CONTENTS

1.Introduction

One of the central questions in neuroscience is how communication in the brain is organized under normal conditions and how this architecture is disrupted by neurological disorders. It has become evident that simple activation studies are no longer sufficient. There is a pressing need to understand the brain as a complex structural and functional network. Interest in brain network research has grown significantly with the advent of modern network theory and increasingly powerful investigative methods, such as high-density EEG, MEG, functional and structural MRI. Contemporary brain network studies have demonstrated that a healthy brain self-organizes into so-called "small-world networks," characterized by a combination of dense local connectivity and critical long-range connections. Additionally, normal brain networks exhibit hierarchical modularity and a connected backbone consisting of interconnected hub nodes. This intricate architecture is thought to arise under genetic control and serves as the foundation for cognition and intelligence. The optimal organization of brain networks is disrupted in neurological diseases in characteristic ways.

1.1. Conceptualizing the Brain as a Network

In 1906, Ramón y Cajal and Camillo Golgi shared the Nobel Prize in Physiology or Medicine. Although they shared the prize, their ideas differed significantly (Jacobson, 1995; Rapport, 2005). Golgi, a proponent of the reticular theory, argued that the brain should be viewed as a large syncytium, or conglomerate, of directly connected neurons. Cajal, on the other hand, used the silver nitrate stain developed by Golgi to interpret his findings in favor of the neuron theory, which proposed that the brain consists of discrete neurons. In a sense, both were correct: the brain is now understood as a vast network of approximately $101010^{10}1010$ neurons, each interacting with around $10410^{4}104$ other neurons, mainly through synapses but also through gap junctions. Gap junctions directly connect the cytoplasm of adjacent cells and can play a role in physiological and pathological synchronization processes.

Alternative views of the brain emphasizing its diffuse and holonomic nature were proposed by Lashley (1923), Pribram and Carlton (1986), and more recently by Nunez (1995). Despite these perspectives, the concept of the brain as a large, complex network of interconnected elements at various scales has become central in modern neuroscience (Nunez, 2010).

1.2. Anatomical and Neurophysiological Evidence for the Network Perspective

The concept of the brain as a complex network is increasingly supported by numerous neuroanatomical and neurophysiological findings. Various types of neurons have been identified, and they connect in characteristic ways, from the level of microcolumns (the smallest functional unit of the brain, containing about 80–100 neurons) and macrocolumns (composed of 60–80 microcolumns; see Buxhoeveden and Casanova, 2002 for a review) to the level of brain regions, lobes, and functional systems. Izhikevich and Edelman (2008) incorporated 22 different neuron types into their whole-brain model.

Advanced techniques are now being used to unravel the precise anatomy at the smallest levels of the brain. Using micro-optical sectioning tomography (MOST), a major breakthrough was achieved in mapping the connections of the mouse brain (Li et al., 2010). Large-scale efforts, such as the Blue Brain Project and the Human Brain Project, are dedicated to describing the microscopic anatomy of the brain (Markram, 2006; Perin et al., 2011; www.humanbrainproject.eu).

At higher resolutions, classical neuroanatomical tracing methods, which successfully demonstrated the network architecture of macaque and cat brains, are now being replaced by modern imaging techniques, particularly high-field MRI combined with DTI (diffusion tensor imaging) and tractography. These methods have revealed large-scale brain connectivity patterns from the voxel level to Brodmann areas (Hagmann et al., 2007, 2008; Gong et al., 2009a).

Since the 1990s, invasive neurophysiological studies in animals have demonstrated communication, primarily through gamma-range synchronization, between widely separated but connected brain regions (Eckhorn et al., 1988; Engel et al., 1991; Gray et al., 1989; König et al., 1995). Many of these findings have since been confirmed using EEG and MEG, demonstrating the existence of functional brain networks, even in a "resting state" (Fell and Axmacher, 2011; Uhlhaas and Singer, 2006).

In a classic review of studies on neurophysiological synchronization, Francisco Varela referred to the brain as the "Brainweb" (Varela et al., 2001). BOLD fMRI (blood oxygen level-dependent) studies confirm the brain's networked nature and provide evidence for the existence of multiple resting-state networks, with the default mode network becoming the most well-known (Damoiseaux et al., 2006). Other resting-state networks or modules correspond to well-established functional systems dedicated to vision, sensorimotor processing, working memory, and attention. To a large extent, structural and functional studies reveal the same complex, and particularly hierarchical, network structure of the brain across multiple levels (Bassett et al., 2008). From a network perspective, anatomical and physiological studies present an increasingly interconnected view of brain organization. Donald Hebb's concept of "synchronous cell assemblies" has evolved from an abstract idea into a neuroanatomical and neurophysiological reality (Hebb, 1949).

1.3. Networks Are Not Enough: The Need for a Theoretical Foundation

Фй=The concept of the brain as a complex structural and functional network, therefore, has a relatively long history and high nominal value given what we know about brain anatomy and neurophysiology. However, the notion of brain networks is too general to be optimally useful for understanding normal and impaired brain physiology unless it is tied to a specific network theory. As Carter Butts noted: "To represent an empirical phenomenon as a network is a theoretical act" (Butts, 2009).

A complex network is more than the sum of the elements that constitute its building blocks; it is also more than the sum of all its pairwise interactions. Complex systems possess emergent properties that require precise mathematical theories for proper understanding (Sporns, 2011a). In this regard, the development of modern network theory in the late 1990s represents an important step forward.

The introduction of powerful new mathematical models of complex networks, such as small-world networks and scale-free networks, has led to widespread and rapidly growing interest in network research across many scientific domains, from physics, communication systems, and transportation to biological and sociological networks (Boccaletti et al., 2006). The advancement of modern network theory has significantly stimulated interest in brain networks and enabled more precise, quantitative studies of the determinants of growth, learning, plasticity, and failures in neural networks.

1.4. Networks in Relation to Complexity Theory

While the network perspective is rapidly becoming a promising approach for understanding the brain's complex nature, it is connected to other scientific domains that deal with complex systems.Cybernetics, information theory, and general systems theory are early examples of attempts to define general mathematical frameworks for complex systems, including neural networks (Shannon and Weaver, 1949; Simon, 1962; von Bertalanffy, 1969; Wiener, 1948). An excellent introduction to modern complexity science can be found in Melanie Mitchell's book *Complexity* (Mitchell, 2009). Modern dynamical systems theory, particularly chaos theory, has significantly influenced our understanding of complex behavior in deterministic yet highly nonlinear systems. These ideas have shaped our concepts of brain function, particularly in relation to the predictability of epileptic seizures (Stam, 2005). Perhaps the most fruitful contribution of nonlinear dynamics has been the development of a general theory of synchronization processes, which is highly relevant to studying the connections between neurons and brain regions (Boccaletti et al., 2002).

1.5. Other important contributions have come from statistical physics and the theory of phase transitions

According to the theory of self-orgaized criticality introduced by Per Bak, complex systems autonomously evolve toward a critical state characterized by power-law distributions (Bak et al., 1987). Currently, there is increasing evidence that such phenomena can also be observed in the brain (Beggs and Plenz, 2003; Werner, 2007). The abundance of complexity theories may suggest a lack of a unifying framework. However, modern network theory is a promising candidate for integrating many emerging concepts in complexity research. Herbert Simon emphasized that complex systems can be viewed as large collections of interacting elements exhibiting hierarchical organization (Simon, 1962).

Modern network theory is based on graph theory as a precise mathematical formalism for describing networks, including their hierarchical organization. Furthermore, it incorporates ideas from probability theory and statistical mechanics to handle the stochastic aspects of large networks, and finally, it includes dynamic systems theory and synchronization to study processes occurring in complex networks (Barrat et al., 2008). Thus, modern network theory represents an appealing and versatile foundation for exploring the organization of complex brain networks.

1.6. The Relevance of Brain Networks to Clinical Neurophysiology

Understanding normal brain function and its disruption in neurological and neuropsychiatric disorders is impossible without considering a network perspective. However, a general, informal understanding of brain networks is no longer sufficient. Modern network theory is beginning to influence our ideas about how brain networks develop, how this development is organized and constrained by genetic and geometric factors, how brain network architecture starts to exhibit universal features such as hierarchical modularity, and how this relates to cognitive function and intelligence. Furthermore, network theory impacts concepts of brain function localization and the global effects of local lesions.

The idea that diverse conditions such as Alzheimer's disease and epilepsy can be explained in terms of "hub failure" clearly illustrates how network science is beginning to influence clinical concepts. Clinical neurophysiology is a medical specialty focused on diagnosing, monitoring, and prognosing clinical neurological conditions using various neurophysiological methods. Modern network theory is particularly relevant to clinical neurophysiology because its two main methods for studying central nervous system function, EEG and MEG, have enormous and barely explored potential for investigating how brain regions interact and how these interactions are disrupted in neurological diseases.

The fact that EEG and MEG directly measure neural activity, rather than indirectly as in the case of fMRI BOLD, is a significant advantage. Combining functional connectivity with modern network theory represents a unique opportunity for clinical neurophysiology. EEG and MEG are not only the most direct tools for measuring brain function; they also provide a window into the brain as a complex, evolving network (Nunez, 2010).

2. Functional Interactions

2.1. Time Series and Brain Function

Understanding how the brain is organized as a functional network requires several elements:

(i) reliable measurement of activity levels in network elements;
(ii) characterization and quantification of connections between network elements;
(iii) integration and analysis of the complete picture of pairwise interactions within the framework of network theory;
(iv) evaluation of the interdependencies between functional and structural levels of the network.

Here, we focus on the first element. The remaining three aspects will be addressed in subsequent sections.

Neurons are the obvious structural and functional building blocks of the nervous system. Neuronal function is reflected in two distinct types of activity:

(i) small fluctuations in the resting membrane potential of dendrites caused by excitatory and inhibitory synapses;
(ii) action potentials along the axon.

A typical pyramidal neuron in the cortex may be covered by 1,000–10,000 synapses, with excitatory synapses predominantly located in the dendritic tree far from the soma, while inhibitory synapses are closer to the cell body. Activation of an excitatory synapse causes a brief depolarization of the membrane potential (excitatory postsynaptic potential, or EPSP), while activation of an inhibitory synapse causes a somewhat larger and longer hyperpolarization of the membrane potential (inhibitory postsynaptic potential, or IPSP).

If the combined effect of all EPSPs and IPSPs on the dendritic tree, determined by spatial and temporal summation, causes the membrane potential near the axon hillock to exceed the threshold, an action potential is generated. This action potential propagates along the axon but also back to the dendritic tree. Neurons influence other neurons via their action potentials, so firing frequency—the number of action potentials per second—is an important parameter of neuronal activity.

A key debate in neuroscience concerns whether relevant information is conveyed solely by firing frequency or also by the precise timing of action potentials. The fact that the exact timing of pre- and postsynaptic neuron firing can influence synaptic plasticity (a concept known as spike-timing-dependent plasticity, or STDP) suggests that timing information may need to be considered (Abbott and Nelson, 2000).

Although neuronal spikes are fundamental for inter-neuronal communication, the most commonly used methods for assessing human brain function, such as EEG, MEG, and fMRI, do not directly measure action potentials. Both EEG and MEG reflect large-scale summed field potentials, which are ultimately caused by excitatory and inhibitory postsynaptic potentials (EPSPs and IPSPs) in cortical, predominantly pyramidal, neurons. Notably, field potentials recorded with EEG and MEG exhibit oscillations across a broad spectrum of frequency ranges, from (sub-)delta to gamma, high-frequency oscillations (HFOs), and ripples (Buzsáki and Draguhn, 2004). The temporal resolution of EEG and MEG is essentially unlimited, which is of interest because it has been shown that both very low-frequency and very high-frequency oscillations have neurophysiological significance (Bragin et al., 2010; Van Someren et al., 2011). The functional significance of oscillatory activity across various frequency ranges has long remained a mystery, and it has even been suggested that these oscillations may be mere epiphenomena (Niedermeyer and Schomer, 2011). However, growing evidence now indicates a phase relationship between oscillatory field potentials and neuronal action potentials (Eckhorn and Obermueller, 1993; Lee et al., 2005). This observation emphasizes that brain oscillatory activity contains information relevant to understanding local and interregional communication.

The BOLD signal reflects the presence of excess oxyhemoglobin in the smallest blood vessels near activated brain regions; it can be regarded as a low-frequency, integrated measure of neuronal impulses with a typical timescale in seconds. Studies combining EEG with fMRI are now beginning to uncover complex relationships between oscillatory band power and BOLD signals (Rosenkranz and Lemieux, 2010). Specifically, a connection has been proposed between the gamma-band oscillation envelope and BOLD time series (Logothetis, 2002).

Time-series methods can be used to analyze recordings of local brain activity via EEG, MEG, and BOLD. The most common method is spectral analysis, which represents signal power as a function of frequency. This approach is particularly useful for identifying oscillatory components of the signal, such as the dominant peak caused by the alpha rhythm and changes in power within specific frequency bands. Activation of specific brain regions is often associated with a decrease or increase in power within a particular frequency band; these changes can be captured using a technique called event-related desynchronization (ERD) or event-related synchronization (ERS) (Pfurtscheller and Lopes da Silva, 1999).

Short-term, non-stationary changes in brain oscillatory activity can also be characterized using evoked or event-related potentials. In contrast to ERD and ERS, which measure induced power changes, evoked and event-related potentials measure only oscillatory changes that are precisely phase-locked to a given event. Another effective method for evaluating non-stationary aspects of oscillatory power is wavelet analysis. Brain oscillatory activity can show correlations across very long timescales.

These correlations can be characterized by spectral analysis, the Hurst exponent, or detrended fluctuation analysis (Benayoun et al., 2010; Linkenkaer-Hansen et al., 2007; Stam and de Bruin, 2004). Finally, non-random structures of oscillatory activity.

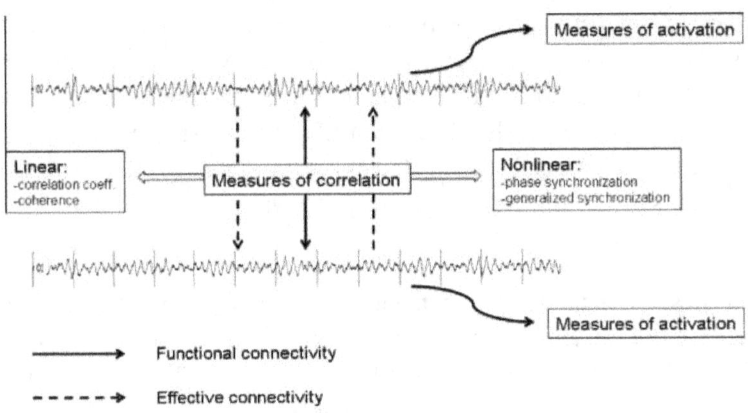

Fig. 2. 1. Schematic Illustration of Time Series Analysis

Activation measures can be derived from individual time series using methods such as spectral analysis.

Correlation measures reflect statistical interdependencies between two time series. These correlations can be bidirectional (functional connectivity) or unidirectional (effective connectivity). Both types of connectivity can be studied using linear methods (e.g., correlation coefficient, coherence) or nonlinear methods (e.g., phase synchronization, generalized synchronization). Two EEG signals recorded at positions O2 and O1 are shown; vertical stripes indicate one-second markers.

Neurophysiological time series analysis can also be characterized using methods derived from nonlinear dynamics. Here, it is assumed that a time series reflects a trajectory in the multidimensional state space of an underlying dynamic system, and this trajectory can be described using measures such as correlation dimension, Lyapunov exponents, and entropy measures (for a review, see Stam, 2005).

2.2. Functional and Effective Connectivity

In the previous section, we discussed how neural or local brain region activity can be measured and characterized using neurophysiological methods and time series analysis. The next step is to consider how this information can be used to infer the connections between neurons and brain regions (Fig. 1). An important concept for understanding connectivity in brain networks is synchronization. Unfortunately, in neurophysiology, synchronization is often used in a rather informal way, referring to an ambiguous notion of the degree of cooperation between neurons. It is frequently assumed that the band power of field potential oscillations reflects these interactions between neurons; however, the band power of EEG or MEG signals recorded at a given electrode or sensor can depend on many factors, and its interpretation in terms of (local) levels of neural synchronization is not straightforward (Daffertshofer and van Wijk, 2011).

In physics, particularly in the theory of dynamical systems, the concept of synchronization has acquired a much more specific and quantitative interpretation, dating back to the pioneering work of the Dutch physicist Christiaan Huygens. Much of the work on synchronization has been based on the notion of phase coupling between pairs of harmonic oscillators (Boccaletti et al., 2002; Rosenblum and Pikovsky, 2003). With the advent of nonlinear dynamics and chaos theory, the concept of synchronization was expanded to include any type of statistical interdependence between dynamic systems, even if they do not exhibit regular oscillations and lack strict phase coupling—so-called generalized synchronization (Rulkov et al., 1995). These advances in synchronization physics have influenced the ability to detect and quantify synchronization in neurophysiological data.

While synchronization in its various manifestations should be considered a fundamental physical concept for understanding correlations between neurophysiological time series, various concepts have also gained popularity in the neuroimaging literature.

Functional connectivity, first introduced by Aertsen et al. (1989), refers to the existence of any statistical interdependence between neurophysiological time series. Initially, this concept referred to recordings of neuronal spikes, but it is now also applied to EEG, MEG, and particularly fMRI (Lowe, 2010; Stevens, 2009). While functional connectivity is a model-free concept, the notion of effective connectivity emphasizes asymmetric causal interactions between neural systems (Friston, 2002).

The concept of effective connectivity is particularly clear in the approach called Dynamic Causal Modeling (DCM), introduced by Karl Friston (Penny et al., 2004). However, it should be emphasized that both effective and functional connectivity can be defined in terms of synchronization theory, i.e., in the language of interacting dynamic systems. This is particularly significant if we aim to achieve a formal understanding of communication processes occurring in complex networks (Arenas et al., 2008).

Numerous time series analysis methods have been developed to characterize the statistical interdependencies between two or more time series of neurophysiological activity. An excellent review is provided by Pereda et al. (2005).

The most important linear measure of correlation between time series is coherence. It can be considered a generalization (with time delay) of the correlation between time series. Coherence describes the strength of the correlation between two time series as a function of frequency; it depends on the consistency of the phase difference as well as the power of the two time series (Nunez et al., 1997). To track correlations in nonstationary signals, coherence can also be based on wavelet analysis (Lachaux et al., 2002).

At least three categories of nonlinear synchronization measures can be distinguished. The first group consists of measures that quantify the consistency of the phase difference between two signals, disregarding the influence of signal amplitude (Rosenblum et al., 1996). Phase synchronization analysis can be based on the Hilbert transform of the data (Mormann et al., 2000) or on wavelet analysis (Lachaux et al., 1999); both approaches are equivalent (Burns, 2004). The second group of measures is based on nonlinear dynamics and quantifies generalized synchronization between attractors reconstructed from the time series (Arnhold et al., 1999; Hu and Nenov, 2004; Pecora and Carroll, 2000; Schiff et al., 1996; Schmitz, 2000). The probability of synchronization is a relatively simple unbiased estimate of generalized synchronization (Stam and van Dijk, 2002; Montez et al., 2006). Finally, there is a group of nonlinear connectivity measures, such as event synchronization and h2, which are not easily characterized (Quian Quiroga et al., 2002; Lopes da Silva et al., 1989).

2.3. Linear and Nonlinear Connectivity Measures

The linear and nonlinear connectivity measures mentioned above are typically symmetric and do not provide information about causality or the direction of influence. One approach to defining effective connectivity is based on Granger causality, originally developed in economics (Granger, 1969). In the context of Granger causality, the future of a time series xxx can be better predicted by considering not only its own past but also the past of another time series yyy. If incorporating information from yyy improves the prediction of xxx, yyy is said to have a causal effect on xxx. A key method for frequency-dependent Granger cau*sality analysis is the Directed Transfer Function (DTF) (Blinowska, 2011).

Connection directionality can also be determined using phase synchronization-based methods, with a notable example being the Phase Slope Index (Nolte et al., 2008). Measures of causal interactions have also been developed within the context of nonlinear dynamic systems (Arnhold et al., 1999; Hu & Nenov, 2004; Pecora & Carroll, 2000; Schiff et al., 1996; Schmitz, 2000). Finally, the nonlinear correlation coefficient h2h^2h2 has also been used to derive a nonlinear directed measure of connectivity (Wendling et al., 2005).

Unlike fMRI, neurophysiological methods for determining connectivity between different brain regions suffer from common-source biases. When activity recorded at two different electrodes or sensors is influenced by a shared underlying source, estimated correlations do not reflect true interactions between distinct neural systems. In EEG, the activity recorded at the reference electrode may also influence estimated correlations between EEG channels (Nunez et al., 1997). These are serious methodological challenges that cannot be easily resolved by performing connectivity analysis in the source space instead of the signal space. While source or Laplacian derivations can mitigate these influences, they do not completely solve the problem and may obscure true long-range interactions. Nunez et al. (1997) proposed a corrected version of coherence to account for volume conduction effects in EEG.

Nolte et al. (2004) suggested using the imaginary part of coherence as a connectivity measure unaffected by volume conduction. However, the drawback of imaginary coherence is that its magnitude is influenced by signal power and the phase delay between channels, making it difficult to interpret increases or decreases. The only definitive conclusion from nonzero imaginary coherence is that volume conduction cannot explain its existence. The Phase Lag Index (PLI) is based on the idea of imaginary coherence but is unaffected by signal amplitude or phase delay magnitude (Stam et al., 2007b). The recently proposed Weighted Phase Lag Index (WPLI) is claimed to be less sensitive to noise but reintroduces dependency on the phase difference magnitude (Vinck et al., 2011). Interestingly, coherence, imaginary coherence, phase coherence, WPLI, and PLI are closely related, as they can all be computed using the Hilbert transform of the data (Stam et al., 2007b).

The availability of so many different synchronization measures raises the question of whether a rational choice can be made among them regarding their performance on real-world data. Several studies have attempted to compare subsets of measures based on their ability to correctly detect synchronization in multidimensional datasets (Ansari-Asl et al., 2006; David et al., 2004; Quian Quiroga et al., 2002a). Unfortunately, the results are inconclusive. The performance of the measures appears to depend on the dataset's characteristics and the method itself. Complex synchronization measures based on nonlinear dynamic system theory require considering many parameters (Montez et al., 2006). Conducting the analysis in the source space does not simplify matters, as each source reconstruction algorithm has its own assumptions that may influence correlations between source signals in unknown ways. The most rational approach at present may be to use multiple methodologies and look for consistent results across them.

2.4. Fragile Binding

Interregional synchronization, or functional/effective connectivity, conveys important information about the healthy brain's functioning. Research has shown that in healthy individuals, the strength of interregional synchronization depends on age. Long-range synchronization is relatively low at birth and increases during development, likely due to the maturation and myelination of long-range association pathways (Barry et al., 2004; Gmehlin et al., 2011; González et al., 2011; Thatcher et al., 2008). The strength of synchronization is influenced by maturation, age, and genetic factors (Chorlian et al., 2007; Posthuma et al., 2005; Van Beijsterveldt et al., 1998). The level of interregional functional connectivity varies across frequency bands and appears to depend on local band power and distance. Some researchers suggest that long-range connectivity is primarily supported by low-frequency synchronization, while short-range connectivity depends on synchronization in the beta and gamma frequency ranges (Von Stein and Sarnthein, 2000). Synchronization strength between different brain areas shows characteristic fluctuations, which may reflect not just noise but the rapid formation and dissolution of functional connections. This dynamic synchronization, even during rest, has been termed "fragile binding" (Stam & de Bruin, 2004). Two distinct models of synchronization dynamics have been proposed: the microstate idea, suggesting that the brain exhibits a sequence of relatively stable states lasting a few hundred milliseconds and linked by abrupt transitions (Lehmann et al., 2006), and a process involving (self-organized) criticality (Beggs & Plenz, 2003; Breakspear et al., 2004; Stam & de Bruin, 2004; Gong et al., 2007). Interregional synchronization also depends on behavioral state and cognition. Sleep induces characteristic synchronization changes across different sleep stages (Ferri et al., 2005). Tasks engaging working memory are associated with increased synchronization, particularly in the theta band and possibly the alpha band (Jensen et al., 2002; Klimesch, 1997; Sarnthein et al., 1998). Gamma synchronization is now considered a crucial neurophysiological mechanism underlying binding, attention, and even consciousness (Dehaene & Changeux, 2011; Fries et al., 2007).

2.5. Excessive Connectivity

Synchronization in the healthy brain is a subtle process characterized by the rapid formation and dissolution of functional connections. This "fragile binding" can be disrupted in two ways: excessive connectivity or disconnection. The most obvious example of excessive synchronization is epilepsy (Lehnertz et al., 2009). At the neuronal level, epileptic phenomena are associated with paroxysmal depolarization shifts (Gorji & Speckmann, 2009). Gap junctions have recently been noted as a critical cause of hypersynchronization in epilepsy (Volman et al., 2011).

Classic interictal and ictal EEG patterns in epilepsy, such as spikes and generalized spike-wave discharges, are often considered to reflect excessive synchronization at both the neuronal and macroscopic levels (Gorji & Speckmann, 2009). However, recent observations of single-neuron activity during human seizures suggest that a model of epilepsy based solely on hypersynchronization may be overly simplistic (Truccolo et al., 2011).

Although certain types of seizures, particularly absence seizures characterized by generalized 3-Hz spike-and-wave discharges, may indeed reflect excessive synchronization compared to pre- and postictal states, this pattern may not hold true for all seizures, especially not for partial seizures. Partial seizures may represent a complex sequence of increases and decreases in synchronization across various frequency ranges at different stages of the seizure. In fact, the highest level of synchronization during partial seizures may only be reached at the very end of the seizure (Schindler et al., 2007).

Preictal changes in EEG synchronization have also become a topic of intense research, particularly since studies by German and French groups suggested the possibility of seizure prediction (Lehnertz and Elger, 1998; Le Van Quyen et al., 2001a; Martinerie et al., 1998). Among all EEG measurements tested for their effectiveness in predicting seizures, interregional synchronization measurements have proven to be the most successful (Mormann et al., 2005). Surprisingly, the preictal state may be characterized by a decrease, rather than an increase, in synchronization (Mormann et al., 2003). It has been suggested that this preictal drop in synchronization may reflect the release of the ictal focus from the inhibitory influence of other brain regions (Le Van Quyen et al., 2001b).

In this regard, the interictal state should be distinguished from the preictal state. There is evidence that synchronization levels during the interictal state are abnormally high, not only compared to the preictal state but also to synchronization levels in healthy individuals. Increased synchronization in the theta range has been described in patients with various types of epilepsy and may predict epilepsy risk even independently of the occurrence of epileptic spikes (Douw et al., 2010b).

2.6. Increased levels of synchronization are not limited to epilepsy

While Parkinson's disease is primarily considered a basal ganglia disorder, elevated interregional synchronization in the alpha range has also been identified in patients with this condition.

The concept of the brain as a large, complex network of interconnected elements has become a dominant paradigm in modern neuroscience (Nunez, 2010). The development of contemporary network theory has significantly fueled interest in brain networks, enabling more precise quantitative research on the determinants of growth, learning, plasticity, and failures in neural networks.

While the network perspective is rapidly emerging as a promising approach to understanding the brain's complex nature, it should be noted that this approach intersects with other scientific fields that deal with complex systems. Complex systems exhibit emergent properties that require precise mathematical theories for proper understanding (Sporns, 2004, 2011a). In this context, the development of modern network theory in the late 1990s represented a significant step forward. The introduction of powerful mathematical models of complex networks, such as small-world networks and scale-free networks, sparked broad and rapidly growing interest in network research across various scientific domains, including physics, communication, transportation, biology, and sociology (Boccaletti et al., 2002, 2006).

Cybernetics, information theory, and general systems theory are early examples of attempts to define common mathematical foundations for complex systems, including neural networks (Shannon CE, Weaver W., 1949; Simon H.A., 1962; von Bertalanffy L., 1969; Wiener N., 1948).

Modern dynamical systems theory, particularly chaos theory, has significantly influenced our understanding of complex behavior in deterministic but highly nonlinear systems. These ideas have shaped our views on brain function, particularly regarding the predictability of epileptic seizures (Stam, 2012). Perhaps the most fruitful contribution of nonlinear dynamics has been the development of a general theory of synchronization processes, which is critical for studying communication between neurons and brain regions (Boccaletti S., Kurths J., Osipov G., Rep et al., 2002; Boccaletti S., Latora V., Moreno Y., et al., 2006).

Herbert Simon emphasized that complex systems can generally be regarded as large sets of interacting elements demonstrating hierarchical organization (Simon H.A., 1962). Modern network theory builds upon graph theory as a precise mathematical framework for describing networks, including their hierarchical organization.

Graphs are essential components of mathematical models in a wide range of scientific and practical fields. They provide a visual representation of relationships between objects or events in complex systems. Many algorithmic problems in discrete mathematics can be formulated as graph-related tasks, such as identifying specific features of a graph's structure, finding a subgraph that meets certain criteria, or constructing a graph with predefined properties.

Every neural network can be interpreted as a separating hyperplane in a multidimensional input space. A set of such planes allows, at least in principle, the construction of arbitrarily complex surfaces. These surfaces can be used to separate objects belonging to different classes.

Network theory also draws on ideas from probability theory and statistical mechanics to address stochastic aspects of large networks and incorporates dynamical systems theory and synchronization to study processes occurring in complex networks (Barrat A., Barthelemy M., Vespignami A., 2008). Thus, modern network theory provides an appealing and versatile foundation for studying the organization of complex brain networks.

Modern dynamical systems theory, particularly chaos theory, has significantly influenced our understanding of complex behavior in deterministic but highly nonlinear systems. These ideas have shaped our views on brain function, particularly regarding the predictability of epileptic seizures (Stam, 2005). Perhaps the most fruitful contribution of nonlinear dynamics has been the development of a general theory of synchronization processes, which is critical for studying communication between neurons and brain regions (Boccaletti S., Kurths J., Osipov G., Valladares DL, Zhou CS., 2002).

Other significant contributions have been made by statistical physics and phase transition theory. According to the theory of self-organized criticality introduced by Per Bak, complex systems evolve autonomously to a critical state characterized by power laws (Bak P., Tang C., Wiesenfeld K., 1987). There is growing evidence that such phenomena may also be observed in the brain (Beggs JM, Plenz D., 2003).

Modern network theory builds upon graph theory as a precise mathematical framework for describing networks, including their hierarchical organization. It also incorporates ideas from probability theory and statistical mechanics to address stochastic aspects of large networks and includes dynamical systems theory and synchronization to study processes in complex networks (Barrat A., Barthelemy M., Vespignami A., 2008). Thus, modern network theory provides an attractive and universal framework for studying the organization of complex brain networks.

In the early 2000s, a group of neuroscientists led by American professor Marcus Raichle (Marcus Raichle, 2010) discovered the resting-state network. This network includes several anatomically distinct but functionally interconnected brain regions: the ventromedial prefrontal cortex, dorsomedial prefrontal cortex, lateral parietal cortex, and the posterior cingulate cortex.

Together with adjacent parts of the precuneus, the entorhinal cortex is often included as part of the network (Raichle Marcus E., 2015). Marcus Raichle suggests that the role of the default mode network (DMN) may be fundamental in the sense that this network maintains a balance between behavioral acts based on more specialized functional systems and a "baseline" state, where a person is not solving any specific tasks but remains awake and ready for action (Raichle Marcus E., 2015). It is assumed that disruptions in the DMN may play a role in various diseases and disorders.

Chapter 1

1.1. Characterization of Material, Methodological Aspects, and Description and Analysis of the Applied Mathematical Apparatus

In the first chapter of the study, EEG recordings were conducted on 14 students with an average age of 20±0.5 years. EEG data were recorded to a computerhard drive using a computerized electroencephalograph with a sampling frequency of 256 Hz in bipolar leads: 1 – forehead-temple, 2 – temple-parietal, 3 – parietal-occipital in the left and right hemispheres during a state of psychosensory rest (eyes closed) for 2 minutes. EEG file analysis was carried out after the experiments using the semi-period analysis algorithm.

Chapters 2 and 3 present the results of EEG analysis of 65 patients diagnosed with intellectual disability (ICD-10 code F70) aged 16–18 years. This primary group was under inpatient examination and treatment at the Communal Non-Commercial Enterprise "Odessa Regional Mental Health Center" of the Odessa Regional Council. The control group consisted of 34 individuals aged 16 to 24 years.

Chapter 2 provides the results of multiple regression analysis to investigate the relationships between EEG rhythms in intellectual disability within the same rhythm, while Chapter 3 addresses the relationships within the same lead. In Chapter 3, EEG analysis results of the control group are presented using multiple regression analysis to study the relationships between EEG rhythms in the control group within the same rhythm and within the same lead.

EEG recording was conducted in a state of relaxed wakefulness with closed eyes using the "Neuron-Spectrum-2" electroencephalograph with a sampling frequency of 500 Hz and a bipolar circular 16-mount configuration. Electrodes were positioned according to the "10-20%" system in 16 cortical areas. EEG recordings followed the international "10%-20%" system from frontal (F3, F4), central (C3, C4), parietal (P3, P4), occipital (O1, O2), anterior temporal (F7, F8), middle temporal (T3, T4), and posterior temporal (T5, T6) cortical zones (odd numbers indicate the left hemisphere, even numbers the right). The bandpass filter ranged from 0.5 to 35 Hz, with a sampling frequency of 500 Hz.

Analysis was performed using periodometric analysis across five standard frequency bands: δ 0.5–4 Hz, θ 4–8 Hz, α 8–13 Hz, β1 13–20 Hz, β2 20–32 Hz.

1.2. Justification for the Use of Multiple Regression Analysis

When conducting a quantitative analysis of EEG, we must first determine what kind of object EEG is: one-dimensional, two-dimensional, or multidimensional. Since EEG is the result of the combined work of at least five EEG rhythm generators (delta, theta, alpha, beta-1, and beta-2), it can be regarded as a multidimensional object (Lobasyuk B.A., 2005).

We live in a three-dimensional space. It is so familiar to us that the properties of spaces with many dimensions often turn out to be unexpected. Nevertheless, it is precisely such spaces that we deal with in pattern recognition (object classification).

The relationships between the amplitude and frequency indicators of EEG have been studied using multiple regression analysis. Because this approach is not generally accepted, we consider it necessary to justify its use.

One approach to identifying relationships between EEG indicators is based on calculating two-dimensional correlation coefficients between the potential fluctuations recorded in different cortical areas. The use of the correlation coefficient as a tool for systemic research can no longer be considered correct. The correlation coefficient $Rx/y=Ry/xR\_$ identifies non-oriented—that is, non-directed—influences from one indicator to another. Moreover, using the correlation coefficient establishes a relation between the concepts of one of the two main types: covariance or causation. There is also the issue of spurious relationships. Only causal relationships have informational value.

When calculating correlation coefficients, the methodology of synthesizing objects of systemic analysis is not employed. Pairwise correlation coefficients do not ensure a description of the properties of brain electric genesis based on the principle of wholeness, "the whole as a whole." According to our understanding, the electrical activity recorded in various regions of the cerebral cortex and subcortical structures is undoubtedly interconnected, and possibly even functions as a function of the electrical activity recorded in other regions of the cerebral cortex and subcortical structures. Therefore, identifying directed—that is, oriented from one cortical region or subcortical structure to another—relationships can contribute to expanding our understanding of the functional state of the central nervous system (CNS).

When considering the brain's electric genesis as a systemic category—that is, as the functioning of a "set of elements that are in certain relationships with each other and with the environment" (L. Von Bertalanffy, 1967)—there arises a need to study the relationships between the individual indicators of electric genesis, which are determined as a result of ECOG (EEG) analysis (between the amplitudes, frequencies, and duration indices of ECOG rhythms in various cortical regions). To address this problem, classical methods of mathematical statistics—multiple regression and correlation analysis—are usually employed.

The use of the correlation coefficient as a tool for systemic research can no longer be considered correct. The correlation coefficient Rx/y=Ry/xR_identifies non-oriented—that is, not directed from one indicator to another—influences. It is now believed that the correlation coefficient (calculated by various methods: the least squares method, Pearson's product-moment correlation, etc.) does not determine the relationship between objects. As Mangheim J.B. and Rich R.K. (1997) write:

"Unfortunately, the correlation coefficient r itself is not easy to interpret. However, one can interpret r2r^2r2 as the degree of reduction in the error in determining Y based on the values of X, i.e. the proportion of Y values that are determined (or can be explained) based on X. r^2 usually They are presented as the percentage share of explained values, while $(1 - r^2)$ is the share of unexplained values. According to Mannheim, J. B. and Rich, R. K., univariate and bivariate analyses never provide a convincing test of hypotheses or theories. In order to test any hypothesis, one must rely on data analysis rather than merely on the formulation of research questions. And this, in turn, requires multivariate analysis—that is, the simultaneous examination of the interrelationships among three or more variables.

Multiple regression analysis is used in cases where one wishes to study the relationships between one independent variable and several dependent variables. The purpose of multiple regression is twofold: (1) to compute the independent impact of changes in the values of each predictor (factor) variable on the outcome variable and to provide an empirical basis for predicting the value of the dependent variable based on the combined influence of the predictors. The general formula for multiple regression is as follows:

$$Y' = a_0 + b_1X_1 + b_2X_2 + \ldots + b_nX_n + e.$$

The equation above is a model of the process under investigation. In multiple regression, the method of least squares works in the same way as in bivariate regression; it involves fitting a line through a set of points—each point representing the values of cases across several variables—in such a way as to minimize the sum of the squared distances from each point to this line.

The value b_i is called the partial regression coefficient; it describes the unique contribution of each independent variable to determining the value of the dependent variable. In other words, the meaning of the regression coefficient in a multiple regression equation is that it indicates how, on average, the outcome variable will change if the corresponding predictor variable increases by one unit while the values of all the other predictors are held constant. In the presence of significant multicollinearity, however, this interpretation of the coefficients becomes impossible. Therefore, when constructing regression models, the effect of multicollinearity should be minimized—for example, by retaining only one variable from each group of closely related predictors.

The efficiency of the regression is assessed by calculating the standard deviation (or standard error) of the regression coefficient, while the adequacy of the regression is determined by computing the coefficient of multiple determination, R^2. This coefficient indicates the extent to which the variations in the dependent variable (expressed as a percentage) are explained by the variations in the set of independent variables. In other words, it is the proportion of the variance in the dependent variable that is accounted for by the independent variables. It also shows how closely the data points cluster around the "line" predicted by our model; it is usually regarded as a measure of the extent to which deviations in the outcome variable can be explained by fluctuations in all the predictors. For example, an R^2 value of 0.57 can be interpreted as indicating that the independent variables in the model explain 57% of the variation in the dependent variable. R^2 ranges between 0 and 1; the closer it is to 1, the more perfect our model.

The basis for testing the significance of a regression lies in the idea of decomposing the variance (scatter) of the outcome variable into factor (explained) and residual (unexplained) components—that is, the portion of the variance explained by the independent factors and the portion that remains unexplained within the model. The measure of the regression's significance is given by the so-called F-statistic—the ratio of the factor variance to the residual variance. The better the regression model, the higher the proportion of factor variance and the lower the proportion of residual variance.

The main tasks addressed by a systems approach are the development and implementation of methods for the analysis and synthesis of objects and the description of their integrated characteristics by representing the objects under study and design as holistic and goal-oriented systems.

1.3. Some Concepts and Definitions in Graph Theory

One possible approach to solving the problem of synthesizing objects in multidimensional research is the geometric interpretation of the equations of multiple linear regression using polycyclic multigraphs (Zykov A. A., 1987) – a mathematical language for the formal representation of concepts related to the analysis and synthesis of structures, systems, and processes, with the aim of their subsequent structural analysis. Graphs represent the most abstract structures encountered in computer science. Any system that assumes the existence of discrete states, or the presence of nodes and transitions between them, can be described by a graph. Any system that assumes the existence of discrete states, or the presence of nodes and transitions between them, can be described by a graph.

A graph is defined as a collection of a finite number of points, called vertices, and lines connecting some pairs of these vertices, called edges or arcs. This definition can be reformulated as follows: a graph is a non-empty set of points (vertices) and segments (edges), both endpoints of which belong to a given set of points. A more rigorous definition is: "A graph $G = (V, E)$ is a combinatorial object consisting of two finite sets: V, called the set of vertices, and a set of pairs of elements from V, i.e. $E \subseteq V \times V$, called the set of edges if the pairs are unordered, and the set of arcs if the pairs are ordered. In the first case, G(V, E) is undirected, and in the second, directed (if $e = (v_1, v_2)$)."

A vertex of a graph is an element of its vertex set. The connections between the nodes of a graph are called edges. An edge of a graph is an element of its edge set. An arc is a directed edge. A graph is called degenerate if it has no edges. Two edges of a graph are said to be parallel if they share the same starting and ending nodes.

Graphs are depicted on the plane as a set of points and the lines or vectors connecting them. In this depiction, the edges may also be rendered as curved lines, and their length does not play any role. A graph G is called planar if it can be represented on the plane in such a way that its edges intersect only at their endpoints.

Vertices of a graph that do not belong to any edge are called isolated. A graph consisting solely of isolated vertices is called a null graph. A graph in which every pair of vertices is connected by an edge is called complete. A graph in which every pair of vertices is connected by a pair of edges is called a complete polycyclic graph. The degree of a vertex is defined as the number of edges incident to that vertex. A graph in which every vertex has the same degree k is called a homogeneous graph of degree k.

Two vertices A and B in a graph are said to be connected (or disconnected) if there exists (or does not exist) a path leading from A to B. A graph is called connected if every two vertices are connected; if there is at least one pair of disconnected vertices, then the graph is called disconnected. A tree is defined as a connected graph that contains no cycles.

Given the above, we have set the goal of developing an algorithm for the systematic analysis of brain electrogenesis using multiple regression analysis and graph theory.

Chapter 2.

The Relationships between EEG Rhythms from Different Leads

Introduction

One of the fundamental problems in electroencephalography is the study of the nature and mechanisms underlying the generation of rhythmic activity. This issue is investigated not only by various neurophysiological methods but also by methods of mathematical modeling. The greatest attention is devoted to the alpha rhythm, which is associated not only with rhythmic but also with cognitive processes (S.A. Isaychev, D.S. Osipova, Yu.M. Koptelov, 2003; E. Basar, M. Shurmann, 1996). The distributed nature of the source of the EEG alpha rhythm has led to the hypothesis that there exist multiple discrete sources of alpha-band oscillations – "alphons" (S.J. Williamson, L. Kaufman, Z.-L. Lu, et al., 1997). It has been suggested that, in a similar fashion, hypothetical generators for the beta-2, beta-1, theta, and delta rhythms exist in the cerebral cortex (B.A. Lobasyuk, 2005). Moreover, it has been shown that the original locations of the generators of EEG frequency rhythms differ significantly along the vertical and anteroposterior dimensions, which, according to the authors, indicates that the EEG rhythms recorded during a single epoch are generated by neural populations located in different regions of the brain (C.M. Michel, D. Lehmann, B. Henggeler, D. Brandeis, 1992). There are also views suggesting that various EEG rhythms are generated by a common or similar source (Albada van S.J., Robinson P.A., 2013). In this regard, the problem of the interrelationship and mutual influence of EEG rhythms recorded from different leads becomes highly relevant. It is also of interest to determine whether the rhythms recorded in different leads are generated by the same generator or by different ones. To answer this question—considering brain electric generation as a systemic category, i.e., as "a set of elements that are in specific relationships with each other and with the environment" (von Bertalanffy)—there arises a necessity to study the relational connections between the individual amplitude and frequency parameters of the EEG rhythms, both within a single lead and across different leads.

Results. In the calculations of the multiple regression coefficients (see Table 2.1; Fig. 2.1):

35

Table 2.1. The number of statistically significant regression coefficients and correlations identified between the amplitudes of EEG rhythms within one lead.

Derivations	Number of coefficients."			
	Amplitudes		Frequencies	
	Regressions	Correlations	Regressions	Correlations
Left				
Forehead–Temple	2	1	2	2
Temple–Vertex	8	3	2	2
Vertex–Occiput	14	8	10	4
Total	24	12	14	8
Right				
Forehead–Temple	6	2	6	3
Temple–Vertex	6	6	4	2
Vertex–Occiput	12	7	6	2
Total	24	15	16	7

Between the amplitudes of EEG rhythms within a single lead, the highest number of regression coefficients was determined in the parietal-occipital lead on the left—14, and on the right—12. When calculating the coefficients of two-dimensional correlation, the highest number of two-dimensional correlation coefficients was also found in these leads—8 and 7, respectively, as well as in the left temporal-parietal lead—6 coefficients.

Between the amplitudes of beta-1 and alpha rhythms, bilateral positive associations were observed in all leads. In the left temporal-parietal (B), left parietal-occipital (C), right temporal-parietal (D), and right parietal-occipital (E) leads, bilateral mutual negative associations were identified between beta-1 and theta rhythm parameters, while bilateral mutual positive associations were found between alpha and theta rhythm parameters (Fig. 1).

In the left parietal-occipital (C), right frontal-temporal (G), and right parietal-occipital (E) leads… [sentence unfinished, please provide the rest if needed].

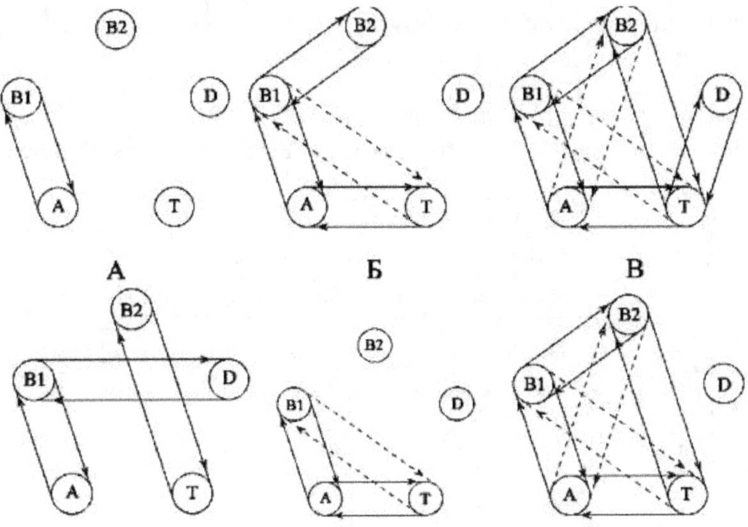

Fig. 2.1. Polycyclic Graphs Describing the Relationships Between EEG Rhythm Amplitude Indicators Within a Single Lead
Designations:
Leads: A – frontal-temporal (left), B – temporal-parietal (left), C – parietal-occipital (left), D – frontal-temporal (right), E – temporal-parietal (right), F – parietal-occipital (right).
EEG rhythms: B2 – beta-2, B1 – beta-1, A – alpha, T – theta, D – delta.

Solid lines connecting graph nodes represent positive regression coefficients, while dashed lines indicate negative regression coefficients from multiple linear regression equations.

Bilateral mutual positive associations were identified between beta-2 and theta rhythm amplitude indicators. All alpha rhythm amplitude indicators in all leads were regression-related to at least one indicator of another EEG rhythm. Notably, the structures of the symmetric polycyclic graphs (Fig. 1, B and D, C and E) were similar.

In the calculation of multivariate regression coefficients (Table 2.1), the highest number of regression coefficients within a single lead was found in the left parietal-occipital lead—10 in total. This lead also showed the highest number of bivariate correlation coefficients—4. It is worth noting that multivariate regression analysis identified a greater number of regression relationships than bivariate correlation coefficients. This may suggest that the relationships between EEG rhythm amplitudes and frequencies are largely nonlinear.

When calculating multivariate regression coefficients (see Table 2.2, Fig. 2.2) between EEG rhythm amplitudes across different leads.

Table 2.2. The number of statistically significant regression and correlation coefficients determined between the amplitudes and frequencies of EEG rhythms across different leads

	Number of coefficients."			
Derivations	Amplitudes		Frequencies	
	Regressions	Correlations	Regressions	Correlations
Left				
Beta-2	8	4	4	4
Beta-1	6	3	8	1
Alpha	20	6	10	3
Theta	4	7	2	9
Delta	2	1	4	3
Total	40	21	28	20

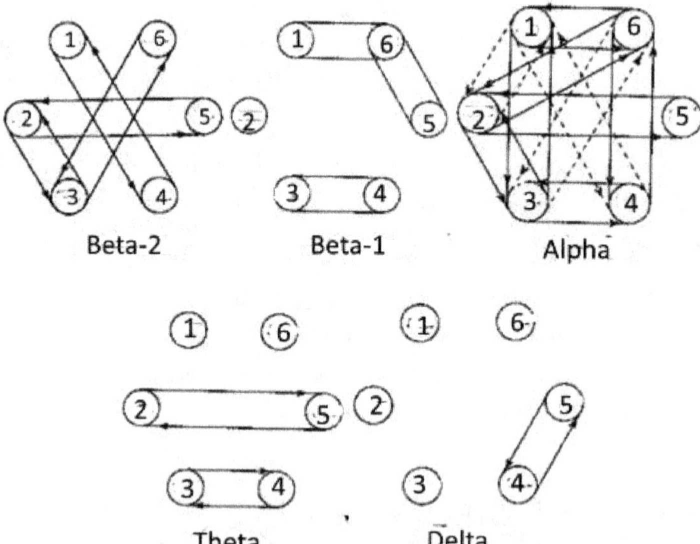

Figure 2.2. Polycyclic graphs describing the relationships between the amplitude indicators of EEG rhythms based on calculations of multiple regression and correlation analysis.
Notations: leads: 1 – right frontal-temporal, 2 – right temporal-parietal, 3 – right parietal-occipital, 6 – left frontal-temporal, 5 – left temporal-parietal, 4– left parietal-occipital.

The greatest number of regression coefficients was determined between the amplitude indicators of the alpha rhythm – 20 coefficients. It should be noted: 1) both positive and negative regression relationships were determined between the amplitude indicators of the alpha rhythm; 2) all amplitude indicators of the alpha rhythm from all six leads were linked by regression relationships. All other amplitude indicators of EEG rhythms, such as beta-2, beta-1, theta, and delta rhythms from different leads, were linked by regression relationships either pairwise – beta-1 and theta rhythms, or in groups of three leads – beta-2 rhythm. When calculating the coefficients of two-dimensional correlation (Table 2, Figure 3), the largest amount…

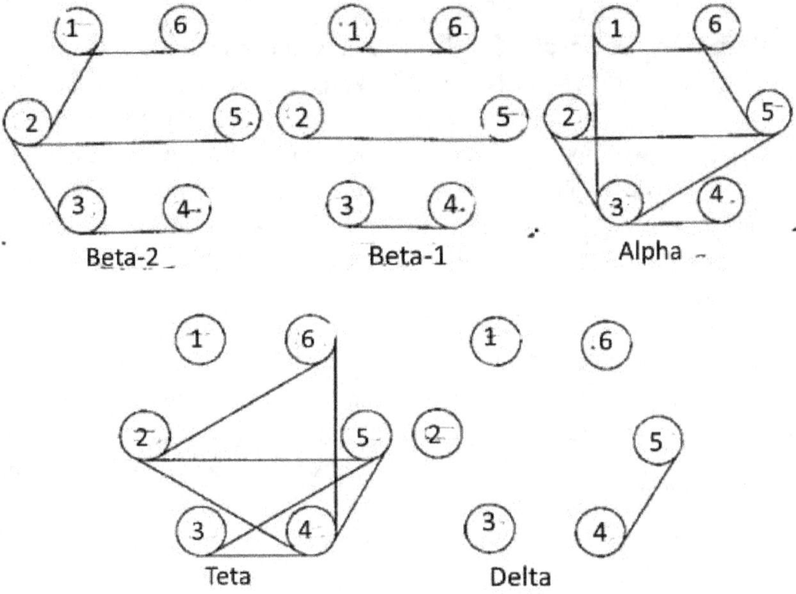

Fig. 2.3. Graphs Describing the Relationships Between EEG Rhythm Amplitude Indicators Based on Two-Dimensional Correlation Analysis
Notation: Same as in Fig. 2.2.

The two-dimensional correlation coefficients were determined between the theta and alpha rhythm indicators, 7 and 6, respectively. Similar to the calculations of multiple regression, in the calculations of two-dimensional correlation coefficients, all amplitude indicators of the alpha rhythm from all six leads were interconnected by correlation relationships. The amplitude indicators of the theta rhythm, except for the theta rhythm amplitude in the right frontotemporal lead, were also interconnected by correlation relationships.

Discussion. A theoretical model of four physical alpha generators located in the upper and lower cortical regions adjacent to the calcarine sulcus in both hemispheres was developed for the human alpha rhythm (R. Cohn, 1948). This model was later refined and supplemented. The localization of at least two separate sources within a 3 cm radius was computed (Lehmann, D., 1972). The most adequate model for describing the distribution of the alpha rhythm across the scalp is believed to be a two-level alpha rhythm generation model with four fixed dipole sources. The first level consists of two basic generators localized in the thalamic reticular nuclei, while the second level is associated with two modality-specific generators localized in the cortical areas corresponding to a specific modality.

Analyzing the polycyclic graph describing the relationships between alpha activity indicators in different leads (Fig. 2.2), both positive and negative relationships can be observed. This may indicate the presence of multiple stationary alpha rhythm generators (at least two) operating at similar frequencies but with different phases. It can also be assumed that alpha activity in different leads is generated by different alpha generators and that the positive and negative relationships found between alpha activity indicators in different leads indicate the presence of control mechanisms within this system of generators.

It is important to note that the regression relationships originating from the graph vertex corresponding to the right temporal-parietal lead had greater absolute values than those directed toward this vertex. This may suggest that the alpha rhythm generator projecting electrical activity to this lead serves as a system-forming element in relation to the other alpha activity generators, whose electrical activity projects to the other analyzed leads. All amplitude indicators of the alpha rhythm from all leads used in constructing the polycyclic graph were interconnected, which may indicate that the analyzed alpha rhythm amplitude indicators belong to a single set of indicators. The obtained results suggest that all possible alpha activity generators are unified into a single whole by control mechanisms.

When calculating the two-dimensional correlation coefficients between the alpha rhythm amplitude indicators of different leads, all analyzed indicators were found to be in correlation relationships. In the right parietal-occipital lead, bidirectional positive mutual influences of the theta and delta rhythms were determined. The facilitating effects of the delta rhythm on theta rhythm generation in the cortex have been demonstrated (Carracedo L.M., Kjeldsen H., Cunnington L., et al., 2013).

The electrical activity of beta-2, beta-1, and theta rhythms appears to be supported by two generators. For the beta-2 rhythm, the electrical activity in the left frontotemporal, right parietal-occipital, right temporal-parietal, and left temporal-parietal leads constitutes the first construct of beta-2 activity, presumably maintained by its generator. The second construct consists of the right frontotemporal and left parietal-occipital leads, where beta-2 activity is likely generated by another generator.

For the beta-1 rhythm, the electrical activity in the right frontotemporal, left frontotemporal, and left temporal-parietal leads forms the first construct of beta-1 activity, presumably supported by its generator. The second construct includes the left and right parietal-occipital leads, which are likely sustained by another beta-1 rhythm generator.

The electrical activity in the left and right temporal-parietal leads, as well as the left and right parietal-occipital leads, in the theta rhythm range, exhibited mutual positive influences (Fig. 2.2). This suggests that EEG electrical activity generation in the theta range is produced by two generators.In the regression analysis of beta-2, beta-1, theta, and delta EEG rhythms, polycyclic multigraphs were not constructed. This may indicate that the generators of these EEG rhythms are multiple.

Chapter 3.

Application of Multiple Regression Analysis for Investigating the Relationships Between EEG Rhythms in Intellectual Disability

Considering brain electrogenesis as a systemic category, i.e., "a set of elements in certain relationships with each other and the environment," it becomes necessary to study the directed connections—relationships formed between individual indicators of electrogenesis, as determined by EEG analysis results (amplitudes, frequencies, indices of EEG rhythm duration). To address this task, classical methods of mathematical statistics can be applied, including multiple regression and correlation analysis. When using this method, all obtained relationships are oriented, meaning they are directed from one object to another and are direct (not indirect).

In recent years, the role of neural networks in the structure of brain activity has become increasingly evident. Interindividual differences at any level (genetic, environmental, etc.) manifest in the organization of neural networks, necessitating a systemic approach for their analysis and understanding. Graph theory, as an example of such a systemic approach, has proven to be a useful tool for network analysis of various neuroimaging data (EEG, MEG, fMRI) (Bullmore E., Sporns O., 2012; Korenkevych D., Chien J.-H, Zhang J., et al., 2013). The systemic approach is based on studying the properties of the whole as a whole. A possible way to synthesize objects in multidimensional research is through the geometric interpretation of multiple linear regression equations using polycyclic multigraphs—a mathematical language for formalized representation of concepts related to the analysis and synthesis of structures, systems, and processes—to enable subsequent structural analysis.

We consider the relationships between EEG rhythms as an important system-organizing factor in electrogenesis. Therefore, by studying the system of oriented relationships—i.e., connections directed from one object to another—it is possible to assess the functional state of EEG and, possibly, approach an understanding of EEG genesis as a system of relationships in the activity of neuronal structures in the brain. According to our understanding, electrical activity recorded in various cortical and subcortical regions is undoubtedly interconnected and may, in fact, functionally depend on electrical activity recorded in other cortical and subcortical regions. Therefore, identifying oriented relationships—i.e., those directed from one cortical or subcortical

43

region to another—can contribute to expanding our understanding of the functional state of the CNS (Lobasyuk B.A., 2010).

EEG coherence was studied in a group of typically developing children and a group of children with mild intellectual disability in a resting state with closed eyes. For resting-state EEG, coherence was higher in children with intellectual disability, and a slight increase with age was observed (Gasser T., Christine Jennen-Steinmetz Ch., 1987).

Besthorn et al. (Besthorn C., Förstl H., Geiger C., et al., 1994) studied 50 patients with dementia and found a decrease in coherence in the theta, alpha, and beta ranges compared to control subjects in central and frontal regions. Their results were consistent with those of Locatelli et al. (Locatelli T., Cursi M., Liberati D., Franceschi M., Comi G., 1998), who showed reduced alpha-range coherence in the left temporo-parieto-occipital region in dementia. Low coherence has been shown to positively correlate with IQ and serve as a predictor of IQ. This suggests that the more complex the neural network and the higher the spatial differentiation, the lower the coherence between different neural pathways (Kanda P.A.M., Anghinah R., Magali Taino Smidth M.T., Jorge Mario Silva J.M., 2009).

The power and coherence of electroencephalography (EEG) in resting state and during a working memory task were studied in patients with mild cognitive impairment. It was found that all power and coherence values in patients with mild cognitive impairment were higher than in the normal control group in both resting state and during working memory tasks. This suggests that mild cognitive impairment may be associated with compensatory processes both at rest and during cognitive tasks. The author suggests that patients with mild cognitive impairment may have impaired normal cortical connections (Zheng-yan Jiang, 2005).

Functional interhemispheric EEG asymmetry is currently recognized as one of the fundamental neurophysiological mechanisms of brain function. A common method for studying functional interhemispheric asymmetry is the fractional linear function (L-R)/(L+R)*100 and coherence analysis. It is of interest to use multiple regression analysis to study interhemispheric asymmetry.

It should be noted that the study of neurodynamic mechanisms in intellectual disability has not been conducted using periodometric EEG mapping analysis. Meanwhile, this computer electroencephalography method is one of the most informative and promising approaches for identifying pathognomonic EEG features.

Thus, the objectives of this study were:

1. To investigate EEG in individuals with intellectual disability using half-period analysis.
2. To examine the relationships between EEG rhythms across all derivations and in all EEG frequency ranges using multiple regression and two-dimensional correlation analysis in comparison with the control group.
3. To study functional interhemispheric asymmetry of EEG rhythm amplitudes in intellectual disability using multiple regression analysis.
4. To compare the results of assessing relationships between EEG rhythms using multiple regression and correlation analysis as well as two-dimensional correlation analysis.
5. To construct graphs reflecting the relationships between EEG rhythms and analyze them.

Own Research

In multiple regression and correlation analysis of the interrelations between the amplitudes of identical rhythms in both hemispheres, the total number of statistically significant regression coefficients in the main group was 1.63 times higher than in the control group (Table 3.1). In the delta and theta ranges, the number of regression coefficients in the main group was lower than in the control group, whereas in the low-beta and high-beta ranges, it was higher. Only in the alpha EEG range was the number of statistically significant regression coefficients the same in both the control and main groups.

The number of two-dimensional correlation coefficients (Table 3.1) between the amplitudes of identical rhythms in both hemispheres was 1.14 times higher in the main group than in the control group. Only in the delta EEG rhythm range was thenumber of two-dimensional correlation coefficients lower in the main group than in the control group; in all other ranges, it was higher.

In multiple regression and correlation analysis of the interrelations between the frequencies of identical EEG rhythms in both hemispheres (Table 2), the total number of statistically significant regression coefficients in individuals with intellectual disability was 1.22 times higher, and the number of two-dimensional correlation coefficients was 1.48 times higher than in the control group.

Table 3.1. Statistically significant regression and correlation coefficients between EEG rhythm amplitude indicators

EEG Rhythms	Number of Coefficients			
	Regression		Correlation	
	(C)	(EG)	(C)	(EG)
Delta	75	82	93	83
Theta	61	104	102	118
Alpha	56	56	95	107
Beta-LF	31	85	75	89
Beta-HF	31	86	58	84
Total	254	413	423	481

Legend:
C – (likely) Control Group
EG – (likely) Experimental Group
Beta-LF – Low-Frequency Beta
Beta-HF – High-Frequency Beta

Thus, both the amplitudes (Table 3.1) and frequencies (Table 3.2) of EEG rhythms in individuals with intellectual disabilities exhibit a greater number of both multiple regression coefficients and two-dimensional correlations.

Table 3.2. Statistically Significant Regression and Correlation Coefficients Between EEG Rhythm Frequency Indicators

EEG Rhythms	Number of Coefficients			
	Regression		Correlation	
	(C)	(EG)	(C)	(EG)
Delta	32	41	44	83
Theta	34	42	84	105
Alpha	29	44	29	66
Beta-LF	32	30	22	40
Beta-HF	38	44	49	45
Total	165	201	228	339

Legend:
C – (likely) Control Group
EG – (likely) Experimental Group
Beta-LF – Low-Frequency Beta
Beta-HF – High-Frequency Beta

To assess lateralization in intellectual disability, calculations of multiple regression and correlation coefficients were performed between the amplitudes of identical EEG rhythms within the same hemisphere—left and right—for right-handed and left-handed individuals in the main and control groups. For this purpose, polycyclic multigraphs were constructed to visualize the relationships between EEG rhythms in right-handed and left-handed individuals from the control group, as well as in individuals with intellectual disabilities in the left (Figure 3.1) and right (Figure 3.2) leads. As seen in the figures, individuals with intellectual disabilities, both right-handed and left-handed, exhibited a greater number of regression relationships than the control group. In both right-handed and left-handed individuals, the most pronounced increase in regression coefficients was observed in the delta, theta, and alpha frequency bands.

In the control group of right-handed individuals (Table 3), calculations of multiple regression coefficients revealed that in the left hemisphere, the number of regression coefficients was higher than in the right hemisphere—28 and 22, respectively—while the number of two-dimensional correlation coefficients was higher in the right hemisphere than in the left—40 and 30, respectively. A greater number of multiple regression coefficients was observed in the delta and alpha rhythms in the right hemisphere, whereas in the theta, low-frequency beta, and high-frequency beta rhythms, more coefficients were found in the left hemisphere.

In the control group of left-handed individuals (Table 3.4), a higher number of regression coefficients was found in the left hemisphere compared to the right—47 and 44, respectively—while the number of two-dimensional correlation coefficients was also higher in the left hemisphere than in the right—80 and 53, respectively. In the delta, alpha, and low-frequency beta bands, a greater number of regression coefficients was identified in the right hemisphere, whereas in the theta and high-frequency beta bands, more were found in the left hemisphere.

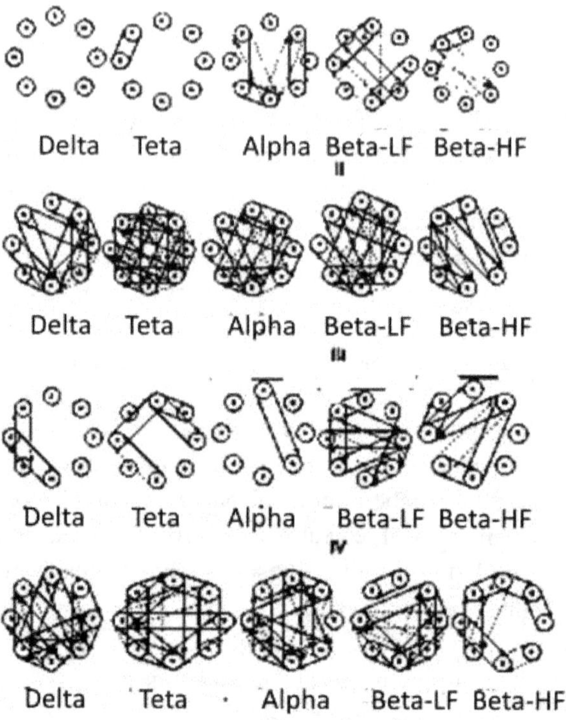

Figure 3.1. Polycyclic Multigraphs Reflecting the Relationships of EEG Rhythms in the Control Group and Individuals with Intellectual Disabilities in the Left Hemisphere
Legend: I – Right-handed, Control, II – Right-handed, Intellectually Disabled, III – Left-handed, Control, IV – Left-handed, Intellectually Disabled,
Electrode placements: 1 – C3–P3 (Central–Parietal), 2 – F3–C3 (Frontal–Central), 3 – F7–T3 (Temporal–Central), 4 – FP1–F3 (Frontal), 5 – FP1–F7 (Frontal–Anterior Temporal), 6 – P3–O1 (Parietal–Occipital), 7 – T3–T5 (Posterior Temporal), 8 – T5–O1 (Temporal–Occipital)

Solid lines indicate **positive influences**, dashed lines indicate **negative influences**.

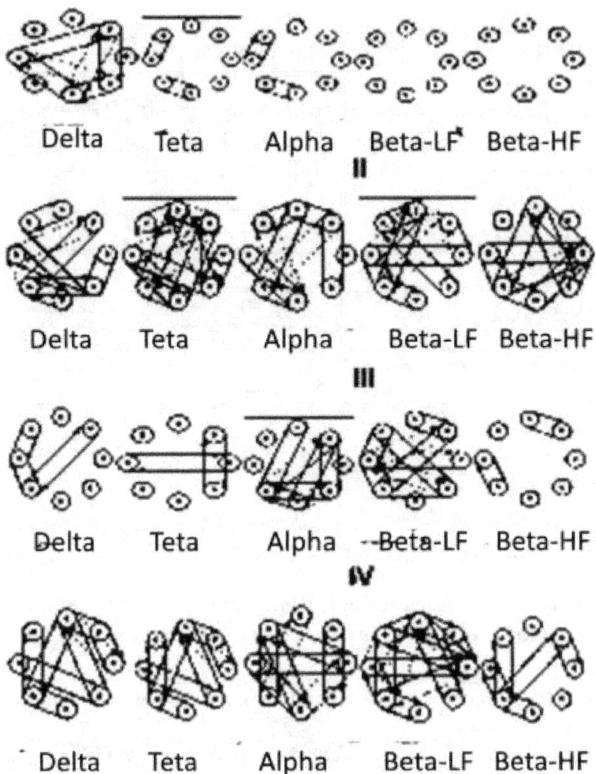

Figure 3.2. Polycyclic Multigraphs Reflecting the Relationships of EEG Rhythms in the Control Group and in Individuals with Intellectual Disabilities in the Right Hemisphere

Legend: I – Right-handed, control group, II – Right-handed, individuals with intellectual disabilities, III – Left-handed, control group, IV – Left-handed, individuals with intellectual disabilities

EEG Leads: 1 – C4–P4 Central–parietal, 2 – F4–C4 Frontal–central, 3 – F8–T4 Temporal–central, 4 – FP2–F4 Frontal, 5 – FP2–F8 Frontotemporal, 6 – P4–O2 Parietal–occipital, 7 – T4–T6 Posterior–temporal, 8 – T6–O2 Temporo–occipital

Solid lines indicate positive influences; dashed lines indicate negative influences.

When comparing right-handed and left-handed individuals in the control group, it was observed that left-handers showed a greater number of regression coefficients in both the left and right hemispheres—1.68 and 2 times more, respectively—compared to right-handers. Additionally, the number of two-dimensional correlation coefficients was 2.66 and 1.33 times higher, respectively (Table 3.3).

Table 3.3. Statistically Significant Regression and Correlation Coefficients Between EEG Rhythm Amplitude Indicators in the Right-Handed Control Group.

EEG Rhythms	Number of Coefficients			
	Regression		Correlation	
	(L)	(R)	(L)	(R)
Delta	0	12	3	2
Theta	10	4	5	12
Alpha	2	6	3	6
Beta-LF	8	0	9	5
Beta-HF	8	0	10	15
Total	28	22	30	40

Legend:

L – Left hemisphere

R-right hemisphere.

Beta-LF – Low-Frequency Beta

Beta-HF – High-Frequency Beta

Table 3.4. Statistically Significant Regression and Correlation Coefficients Between EEG Rhythm Amplitude Indicators in the Control Group of Left-Handed Participants

EEG Rhythms	Number of Coefficients			
	Regression		Correlation	
	(L)	(R)	(L)	(R)
Delta	4	6	10	10
Theta	15	4	25	19
Alpha	2	14	18	8
Beta-LF	14	16	5	7
Beta-HF	12	4	22	9
Total	47	44	80	53

Legend:

L – Left hemisphere

R-right hemisphere.

Beta-LF – Low-Frequency Beta

Beta-HF – High-Frequency Beta

In mentally retarded right-handed individuals (Table 3.5), as in the control group, a greater number of regression coefficients were determined in the left hemisphere than in the right (131 and 102, respectively), while a greater number of two-dimensional correlation coefficients were found in the right hemisphere than in the left (63 and 42, respectively).

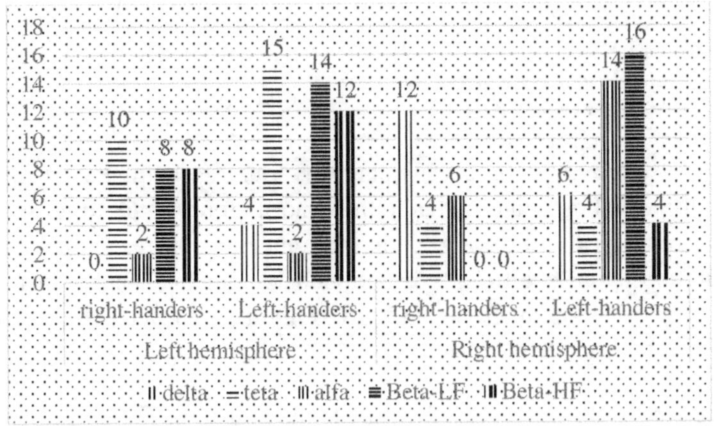

Figure 3.3 Statistically Significant Regression Coefficients Between EEG Rhythm Amplitudes in Right-Handed and Left-Handed Participants of the Control Group

Legend: Left – Left Hemisphere, Right – Right Hemisphere.

In the delta, theta, alpha, and low-frequency beta ranges, more regression coefficients were observed in the left hemisphere than in the right. In the low-frequency beta range, more coefficients were observed in the right hemisphere.

Table 3.5. Statistically Significant Regression and Correlation Coefficients Between EEG Rhythm Amplitude Indicators in Mentally Retarded Right-Handed Individuals

EEG Rhythms	Number of Coefficients			
	Regression		Correlation	
	(L)	(R)	(L)	(R)
Delta	22	18	10	17
Theta	38	30	24	18
Alpha	28	16	0	0
Beta-LF	28	22	0	19
Beta-HF	15	16	8	9

EEG Rhythms	Number of Coefficients			
	Regression		Correlation	
	(L)	(R)	(L)	(R)
Total	131	102	42	63

Legend:
L – Left hemisphere
R-right hemisphere.
Beta-LF – Low-Frequency Beta
Beta-HF – High-Frequency Beta

The number of regression coefficients was found to be higher in intellectually disabled right-handed individuals than in the control group—**1.68 times higher** in the left hemisphere and **1.64 times higher** in the right hemisphere. The number of two-dimensional correlation coefficients in individuals with intellectual disabilities was also higher than in the control group—**1.4 times higher** in the left hemisphere and **1.56 times higher** in the right hemisphere.

In intellectually disabled left-handed individuals (Table 3.6), similar to intellectually disabled right-handed individuals, a greater number of regression coefficients were identified in the left hemisphere than in the right (**116 and 82**, respectively). Conversely, a greater number of two-dimensional correlation coefficients were observed in the right hemisphere than in the left (**109 and 101**, respectively).

Across all EEG frequency ranges, more regression coefficients were found in the left hemisphere than in the right.

Table 3.6. Statistically significant regression and correlation coefficients between EEG rhythm amplitude indicators in intellectually disabled left-handed individuals

EEG Rhythms	Number of Coefficients			
	Regression		Correlation	
	(L)	(R)	(L)	(R)
Delta	28	16	13	22
Theta	22	18	21	26
Alpha	26	16	25	18
Beta-LF	26	25	21	21
Beta-HF	14	7	21	22

EEG Rhythms	Number of Coefficients			
	Regression		Correlation	
	(L)	(R)	(L)	(R)
Total	116	82	101	109

Legend:
L – Left hemisphere
R-right hemisphere.
Beta-LF – Low-Frequency Beta
Beta-HF – High-Frequency Beta

As with mentally retarded right-handers, mentally retarded left-handers showed a higher number of regression coefficients in the left hemisphere—2.46 times more— and in the right hemisphere—1.86 times more—compared to the corresponding control group. The number of two-dimensional correlation coefficients was also higher in the group of mentally retarded left-handers than in the control group—1.26 times more in the left hemisphere and 2.06 times more in the right hemisphere.

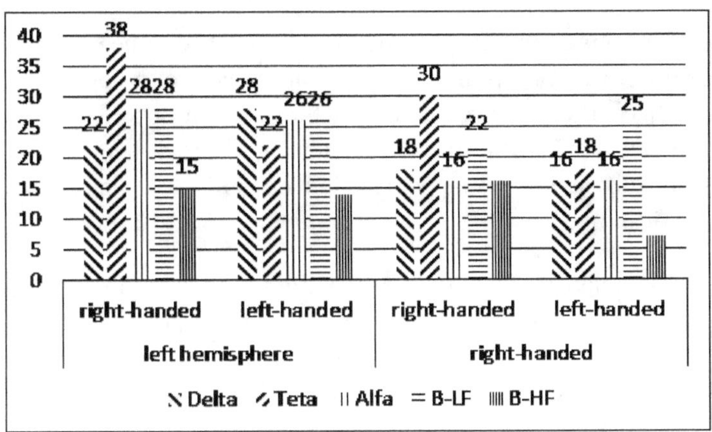

Figure 3.4. Statistically Significant Regression Coefficients Between EEG Rhythm Amplitudes in Right-Handed and Left-Handed Individuals with Intellectual Disabilities.
Designations: Same as in Figure 3.3.

Comparing right-handed and left-handed individuals with intellectual disabilities, it can be noted that, unlike in the control group, the number of statistically significant regression coefficients in left-handers was lower than in right-handers. However, the number of correlation coefficients, as in the control group, was higher in left-handers.

Discussion. In the multiple regression and correlation analysis of the mutual influences of amplitudes of identical rhythms and frequencies in both hemispheres in individuals with intellectual disabilities, more multiple regression coefficients and two-dimensional correlation coefficients were identified. This may be due to the formation of compensatory neurophysiological mechanisms in individuals with intellectual disabilities (Zheng-yan Jiang, 2005).

The highest number of regression coefficients in the control group was found in the delta range, while in the main group, it was in the theta range. The highest number of correlation coefficients, in both the control and the main groups, was identified in the theta range. In all EEG ranges, except for the alpha rhythm range, the number of multiple regression coefficients was higher in individuals with intellectual disabilities than in the control group. In the alpha rhythm range, the number of multiple regression coefficients was the same in both groups. This may indicate that the system generating the alpha rhythm in individuals with intellectual disabilities is more severely damaged than the systems generating other EEG rhythms and becomes incapable of forming compensatory responses.

When calculating multiple regression and two-dimensional correlation coefficients between EEG rhythm amplitudes in the control group of right-handers, more regression coefficients were found in the left hemisphere, while more two-dimensional correlation coefficients were found in the right hemisphere. This may indicate that different mathematical functions correspond to different neurophysiological functions.

The highest number of multiple regression coefficients in right-handers was identified in the theta rhythm range in the left hemisphere and in the delta rhythm range in the right hemisphere. The highest number of two-dimensional correlation coefficients, in both the left and right hemispheres, was identified in the low-frequency beta range.

In the control group of left-handers, both the number of multiple regression coefficients and two-dimensional correlation coefficients were higher than in the control group of right-handers.

Considering that an increase in the number of correlation connections between different EEG components reflects an overall increase in cortical tone, while a decrease reflects a reduction in tone, it can be assumed that left-handers have a higher cortical tone compared to right-handers.

When studying coherence functions in healthy right-handers during a state of calm wakefulness, most studies note the advantage of the degree of alpha rhythm synchronization as the most informative criterion of functional connectivity of cortical structures in the left hemisphere.

Along with this, there are also reports that right-handers exhibit higher coherence values in the frontal areas of the right hemisphere for the alpha and beta-2 frequency bands during interhemispheric analysis and for the delta and theta bands during intrahemispheric analysis (Tucker M., Stenslie C.E., Randy S. et al., 1981).

Flor Henry and colleagues (1982) found that right-handers, in a state of relaxed wakefulness, showed higher intrahemispheric coherence values for the beta-2 band in the right hemisphere when assessing intrahemispheric coherence using the conventional method, i.e., by comparing coherence in homologous pairs within each hemisphere.

In our studies, a greater number of regression coefficients, in both right- and left-handers from the control group, were found in the left hemisphere. A higher number of two-dimensional correlations in right-handers were identified in the right hemisphere, while in left-handers, they were found in the left hemisphere.

When calculating correlation coefficients, strictly linear relationships are determined, whereas multiple regression coefficients account for both linear and nonlinear relationships. It can be assumed that brain structure interactions are realized through both linear and nonlinear functions.

Research on EEG functional connectivity related to handedness is limited and poorly comparable. For example, using only two pairs of electrodes (Fz-P3 and Fz-P4) for interhemispheric EEG coherence in the alpha band, opposite changes were observed between resting conditions and spatial mental tasks (Shaw J.C., O'Connor K.P., Ongley C., 1977).

When calculating multiple regression and two-dimensional correlation coefficients for rhythm amplitudes in left-handers, more multiple regression and two-dimensional correlation coefficients were found in the left hemisphere than in the right.

In left-handers, the highest number of regression coefficients in the left hemisphere was observed in the theta and low-frequency beta bands, while in the right hemisphere, it was in the low-frequency beta band.

In the group of mentally retarded right-handers, more regression coefficients were found in the left hemisphere than in the right, and more two-dimensional correlation coefficients were identified in the right hemisphere than in the left. These patterns were also observed in the control group of right-handers. This may indicate the preservation of neurophysiological mechanisms supporting both linear and nonlinear relationships in the mentally retarded subjects.

The highest number of regression coefficients in the group of mentally retarded right-handers was found in the theta band in both hemispheres. The highest number of correlation coefficients was found in the theta band in the left hemisphere and in the low-frequency beta band in the right hemisphere. In the control group of right-handers, the highest number of regression coefficients was found in the theta band in the left hemisphere and in the delta band in the right. The highest number of two-dimensional correlation coefficients was observed in the high-frequency beta band. The observed differences may indicate a special functional significance of the theta rhythm in neurophysiological support in mentally retarded subjects.

In the group of mentally retarded left-handers, the highest number of regression coefficients was found in the delta rhythm range in the left hemisphere and in the low-frequency beta rhythm range in the right hemisphere. The highest number of two-dimensional correlation coefficients was found in the alpha range in the left hemisphere and in the theta range in the right. In the control group of left-handers, the highest number of regression coefficients was found in the theta range in the left hemisphere, similar to the control group of right-handers, and in the low-frequency beta range in the right hemisphere. The highest number of two-dimensional correlation coefficients was observed in the theta range in both hemispheres and in the right hemisphere. The observed differences may indicate a special role of alpha rhythm synchronization in individuals with intellectual disabilities for the formation of compensatory mechanisms.

In the group of left-handed individuals with intellectual disabilities, the number of regression coefficients was lower than in right-handed individuals, but the number of correlation coefficients was higher. The observed increase in correlation coefficients may indicate an increased cortical tone in left-handed individuals with intellectual disabilities compared to right-handed individuals with intellectual disabilities, and the mechanism of this increased tone is realized through linear functions.

Conclusions:

1. Among individuals with intellectual disabilities, a greater number of multiple regression coefficients and two-dimensional correlation coefficients were identified in the EEG rhythm amplitude and frequency indicators. This may be due to the formation of a system of compensatory neurophysiological mechanisms in individuals with intellectual disabilities.
2. In the control group, both multiple regression coefficients and two-dimensional correlation coefficients were greater in left-handed individuals than in right-handed individuals. This suggests that, compared to right-handed individuals, left-handed individuals may have increased cortical tone.
3. A greater number of regression coefficients, in both right-handed and left-handed individuals, was found in the left hemisphere. A greater number of two-dimensional correlation coefficients was observed in the right hemisphere for right-handed individuals and in the left hemisphere for left-handed individuals. This suggests that the calculation of multiple regression and two-dimensional correlation coefficients reveals different aspects of electrogenesis.
4. The topographical differences in the number of identified multiple regression and two-dimensional correlation coefficients suggest that brain structure interactions are realized through both linear and nonlinear functions.

Chapter 4.

Application of Multiple Regression Analysis to Investigate the Relationships Between EEG Rhythm Amplitudes Within a Single Lead in Intellectual Disability

The modern stage of scientific development is characterized by the creation of algorithms for analyzing the activity of complex multi-level systems, including the brain of animals and humans. The primary focus of these studies is not material objects per se, but the connections and relationships that form the systems of the world around us.

One of the fundamental problems of electroencephalography (EEG) is the study of the nature and mechanisms of rhythmic activity generation. This problem is addressed not only through various neurophysiological methods but also through mathematical modeling approaches (Lobasyuk B.A., 2010; 2016). The greatest attention is paid to the alpha rhythm, which is associated not only with rhythmic but also with cognitive processes (Andersson S.A., Holmgren E., 1975; Basar E., 1998).

Several theories regarding the origin and localization of alpha rhythm generators are considered. The pacemaker theory, presented by P. Andersen and his colleagues, is based on the localization of the central alpha rhythm generation mechanism in thalamic nuclei, which influence neuronal activity in corresponding cortical areas (Andersen P., Andersson S.A., 1974; Andersson S.A., Holmgren E., 1975).

The model of cortical and thalamic generators, proposed by F. Lopes da Silva and colleagues (Lopes da Silva F.H., van Lierop T.H.M.T., Schrijer C.F.M., Storm van Leeuwen W., 1973), is based on the existence of relatively independent generators located both in the thalamic nuclei and the cortex.

The theory of Basar E. (Andersson S.A., Holmgren E., 1975; Basar E., 1998) posits the existence of multiple multifunctional generators of alpha rhythm selectively distributed throughout the brain, forming a diffusely distributed alpha system.

Previously, using multiple regression analysis, we identified mutually oriented (vector) interactions between the amplitude indicators of electrocorticographic (ECoG) rhythms. These results are consistent with the general understanding of the forebrain functioning as a unified whole. The distributed nature of the alpha rhythm source in the electroencephalogram (EEG) led to the hypothesis that multiple discrete sources of alpha-band oscillations—"alphons"—exist (Williamson S.J., Kaufman L., Lu Z.-L., et al., 1997). We further hypothesized that similar hypothetical generators might exist in the cerebral cortex for beta-2, beta-1, theta, and delta rhythms (Lobasyuk B.A., 2005; 2010).

There are concepts suggesting that dynamic functional connections between different cortical and subcortical structures should play a leading role in brain function (Weiss S., Rappelsberger P., 1998).

According to modern views, EEG rhythms are generated by corresponding generators. By studying the connectivity (mutual influence) of the amplitudes of various EEG rhythms, we are essentially examining the connectivity of different EEG rhythm generators. The presence of relationships between the amplitudes of EEG rhythms within a single lead indicates the existence of control mechanisms between them. The literature lacks information on the functional connectivity (mutual influence) between individual EEG rhythms.

It has been shown that the original locations of EEG frequency rhythm generators differed significantly in vertical and anteroposterior dimensions. The authors believe this indicates that EEG rhythms recorded during a single EEG epoch are generated by neuronal populations located in different brain regions (Michel C.M., Lehmann D., Henggeler B., Brandeis D., 1992). Therefore, by studying the relationships (mutual influence) of amplitudes of different EEG frequency bands, one can gain insight into the relationships between neuronal populations located in various brain regions and generating EEG rhythms.

There are also views suggesting that different EEG rhythms may be generated by a common or similar source (Albada van S.J., Robinson P.A., 2013).

Michel C.M. (1992) studied the localization of delta-, theta-, alpha-, and beta-frequency EEG sources using dipole approximation, fast Fourier transform, and three-dimensional dipole modeling. The analysis showed that, in subjects, the locations of EEG frequency band sources varied significantly along vertical and anteroposterior dimensions. The delta source was the deepest and most anterior, theta was more posterior and less deep, alpha was the most posterior and highest in vertical dimension, beta-1 was deeper and slightly anterior to alpha, and beta-2 was even earlier and deeper than beta-1. Thus, the depth of the source location was not linearly related to temporal frequency. The sources of all five bands were oriented in the sagittal direction. The results indicate that different EEG frequency bands during a given EEG epoch are generated by neuronal populations in different brain regions.

Studies by Isaichev S.A., Derevyankin V.T., Koptelov Yu.M., and Sokolov E.N. (2001) identified two sources of alpha rhythm generation located in the thalamic structures of the brain, operating within a narrow frequency range with maximum resonance response frequencies of 10.1 and 10.5 Hz.

It has been shown that each delta, theta, alpha, and beta rhythm of traditional EEG arises from several anatomically distinct brain structures. The results of these studies imply the presence of distributed regional sources of brain rhythms and support the view that during preparatory attention, modulation of brain sources generating alpha and beta rhythms occurs (Marco-Pallarés J., Grau C., 2006).

In recent years, the role of neural networks in the structure of brain activity has become increasingly evident (Pardalos P.M., Du D.-Z., Graham R.L., 2013).

Interest in network science has increased significantly over the past decades. Network models have been recognized as a crucial tool for analyzing the dynamics of complex systems. Networks appear to be widespread and have certain special properties that make them particularly suitable for modeling the brain (Korenkevych D., Chien J.H., Zhang J., 2013).

The formation of neural networks is possible based on systems analysis. Graph theory, as an example of such a systemic approach, proves to be a useful tool for network analysis of various neuroimaging data (EEG, MEG, fMRI) (*The economy of brain network organization – Nature Reviews Neuroscience*, 2012).

Therefore, constructing polycyclic multigraphs that visualize directed (i.e., from one EEG frequency range amplitude indicator to another) relational connections (semantic cases) can help expand our understanding of the functional state of the central nervous system (CNS).

The aim of our study was to:

1. Investigate EEG in individuals with intellectual disabilities using half-period analysis.

2. Study the relationships between EEG amplitudes of different frequency ranges within a single lead and across all leads in individuals with intellectual disabilities compared to controls, using multiple regression analysis.
3. Construct polycyclic multigraphs reflecting the relationships between EEG rhythms within each lead and analyze them.
4. Examine functional interhemispheric asymmetry of EEG rhythm amplitudes in individuals with intellectual disabilities using multiple regression analysis.

Own research and discussion: During multiple regression analysis of amplitude relationships...

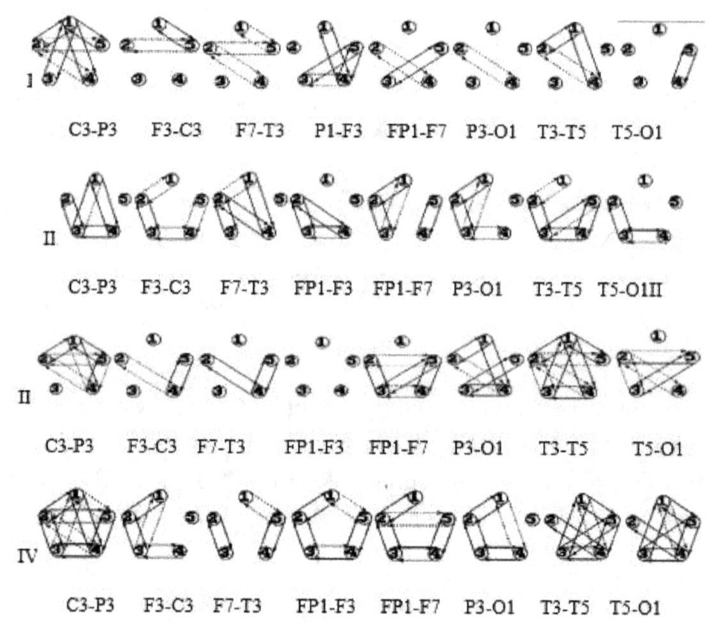

Figure 1. Polycyclic Multigraphs Reflecting the Relationships Between EEG Rhythm Amplitudes Within a Single Lead in the Control Group and in Individuals with Intellectual Disabilities in the Left Hemisphere

Legend: I – Right-handed, control, II – Right-handed, intellectually disabled, III – Left-handed, control, IV – Left-handed, intellectually disabled

Leads: C3–P3: Central-parietal, **F3–C3**: Frontal-central, **F7–T3**: Temporal-central, **FP1–F3**: Frontal, **FP1–F7**: Frontotemporal, **P3–O1**: Parietal-occipital, **T3–T5**: Posterior-temporal, **T5–O1**: Temporo-occipital,

EEG Rhythms: 1 – Delta, 2 – Theta, 3 – Alpha4 – Beta (low-frequency), 5 – Beta (high-frequency)

Line Types: Solid lines: Positive influences, **Dashed lines:** Negative influences

The analysis of EEG rhythms across various frequency ranges within a single lead (Figures 4.1, 4.2, 4.3) revealed that, under normal conditions, right-handed individuals exhibit 1.4 times more regression relationships in the left hemisphere than in the right hemisphere. In left-handed individuals under normal conditions, a greater number of relationships—1.16 times more—are observed in the right hemisphere.

It is noteworthy that the number of relationships in left-handed individuals was higher than in right-handed individuals: 1.53 times more in the left hemisphere and 2.47 times more in the right hemisphere.

In individuals with intellectual disabilities, right-handed subjects showed 1.43 times more relationships in the right hemisphere than in the left. Among left-handed individuals with intellectual disabilities, a slightly higher number of relationships—1.02 times more—was observed in the left hemisphere than in the right (Figures 4.1, 4.2, 4.3).

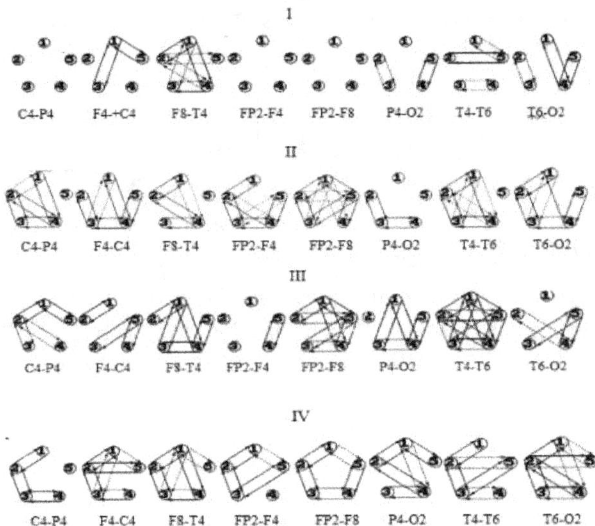

Figure 4.2. Polycyclic Multigraphs Reflecting the Relationships Between EEG Rhythm Amplitudes in the Control Group and Individuals with Intellectual Disabilities in the Right Hemisphere

Legend: I – Right-handed, control, II – Right-handed, intellectually disabled, III – Left-handed, control, IV – Left-handed, intellectually disabled

Electrode placements: C4–P4: Central-parietal, **F4–C4**: Frontal-central, **F8–T4**: Temporal-central, **FP2–F4**: Frontal, **FP2–F8**: Fronto-temporal, **P4–O2**: Parieto-occipital, **T4–T6**: Posterior-temporal, **T6–O2**: Temporo-occipital

EEG Rhythms: 1 – Delta, 2 – Theta, 3 – Alpha, 4 – Beta (low-frequency), 5 – Beta (high-frequency)

Line types: Solid lines – Positive influences, Dashed lines – Negative influences

In individuals with intellectual disabilities, the number of regression relationships was higher than under normal conditions: for right-handers, 1.43 times more in the left hemisphere and 2.87 times more in the right hemisphere; for left-handers, 1.31 times more in the left hemisphere and 1.11 times more in the right hemisphere.

The highest number of connections for right-handers under normal conditions in the left hemisphere was recorded at the C3-P3 (central-parietal) lead — 12, and in the right hemisphere at the F8-T4 (temporal-central) lead — also 12. The lowest number of connections for right-handers under normal conditions in the left hemisphere was recorded at the P3-O1 (parietal-occipital) and T5-O1 (temporal-occipital) leads — two connections each.

The highest number of connections for left-handers under normal conditions in the left hemisphere was recorded at the T3-T5 (posterior-temporal) lead — 16, and in the right hemisphere at the T4-T6 (posterior-temporal) lead — 20. The lowest number of connections for left-handers under normal conditions in the left hemisphere was recorded at the FP1-F3 (frontal) lead — 0, and in the right hemisphere at the FP2-F4 (frontal) lead — 2.

For individuals with intellectual disabilities, the highest number of connections for right-handers in the left hemisphere was recorded at the T3-T5 (posterior-temporal) lead — 10, and in the right hemisphere at the FP2-F8 (anterior-temporal) lead — 18, indicating higher activation in these regions. The lowest number of connections for right-handers with intellectual disabilities in the left hemisphere was recorded at the T5-O1 (temporal-occipital) lead — 4, and in the right hemisphere at the P4-O2 (parietal-occipital) lead — 4, indicating lower activation in these regions.

For left-handers with intellectual disabilities, the highest number of connections in the left hemisphere was recorded at the C3-P3 (central-parietal) lead — 16, and in the right hemisphere at the T6-O2 (temporal-occipital) lead — 14. The lowest number of connections for left-handers with intellectual disabilities in the left hemisphere was recorded at the F7-T3 (temporal-central) lead — 6, and in the right hemisphere at the C4-P4 (central-parietal) lead — 6.

Under normal conditions, for right-handers, no alpha rhythm amplitude relationships from other EEG rhythm amplitudes were detected in the following leads in the left hemisphere: F3-C3 (frontal-central), F7-T3 (temporal-central), P3-O1 (parietal-occipital), T3-T5 (posterior-temporal), and T5-O1 (temporal-occipital). In the right hemisphere under normal conditions, no alpha rhythm amplitude relationships were detected at the C4-P4 (central-parietal), FP2-F4 (frontal), and FP2-F8 (anterior-temporal) leads.

For left-handers under normal conditions, no alpha rhythm amplitude relationships were detected in the left hemisphere at the C3-P3 (central-parietal), F3-C3 (frontal-central), F7-T3 (temporal-central), and FP1-F3 (frontal) leads. In the right hemisphere, no alpha rhythm amplitude relationships were detected only at the FP2-F4 (frontal) lead.

In individuals with intellectual disabilities (both right- and left-handers), alpha rhythm amplitude relationships from other EEG rhythm amplitudes were detected in both hemispheres.

In the delta range under normal conditions, right-handers showed more regression relationships in the left hemisphere, and left-handers in the right hemisphere. In individuals with intellectual disabilities, both right- and left-handers showed more regression relationships in the right hemisphere.

In the theta range under normal conditions, both right- and left-handers showed more regression relationships in the left hemisphere, while individuals with intellectual disabilities (both right- and left-handers) showed more regression relationships in the right hemisphere.

In the alpha rhythm range under normal conditions, both right- and left-handers showed more regression relationships in the right hemisphere. Individuals with intellectual disabilities showed more regression relationships overall.

It was determined in the right hemisphere, while in left-handers, the number of regression connections-relations in both hemispheres was the same.

In the beta low-frequency range, under normal conditions, right-handers showed a greater number of regression connections-relations in the left hemisphere, while left-handers showed more in the right hemisphere. Among intellectually disabled right-handers, a greater number of regression connections-relations were observed in the right hemisphere, whereas in left-handers, they were in the left hemisphere.

In the beta high-frequency range, under normal conditions, right-handers exhibited a greater number of regression connections-relations in the left hemisphere, while left-handers exhibited more in the right hemisphere. Among intellectually disabled right-handers, a greater number of regression connections-relations were found in the right hemisphere, and in left-handers, in the left hemisphere.

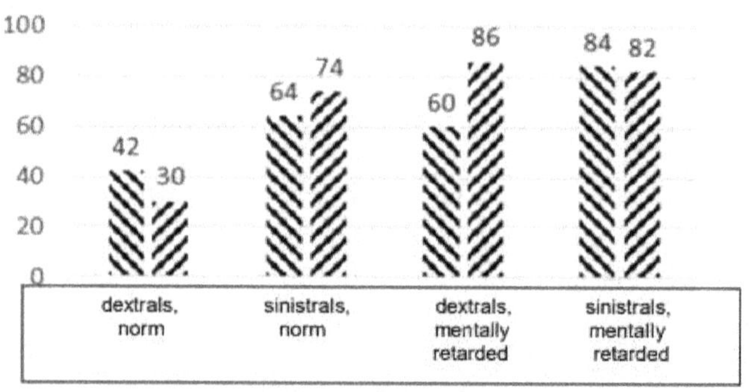

Fig. 3. Statistically significant regression coefficients reflecting the relationship between the amplitudes of EEG rhythms determined within one lead. Notation: Sinistral -Sinistral Hemisphere, Dextral-Dextral Hemisphere

Table 4.1. Statistically significant regression coefficients between the amplitud4.es of EEG rhythms in frequency ranges within one lead EEG rhythms Norm Mentally

EEG rhythms	Norm				Mentally retarded			
	Dextrals		Sinistrals		Dextrals		Sinistrals	
	Hemispheres							
	Sinistral	Dextral	Sinistral	Dextral	Sinistral	Dextral	Sinistral	Dextral
Delta	18	12	18	30	20	34	32	38
Theta	20	12	32	24	30	36	36	40
Alpha	6	12	20	26	36	40	36	36
Beta low frequency	22	14	32	34	26	42	40	26
Beta high frequency	20	12	26	32	8	16	26	24

Table 4.2. Coefficients of interhemispheric asymmetry of the number of coefficients of multiple regression between the amplitudes of EEG rhythms

EEG rhythms	Norm		Mentally retarded	
	Dextrals	Sinistrals	Dextrals	Sinistrals
Delta	20,00	-25,00	-25,93	-8,57
Theta	25,00	14,29	-9,09	-5,26
Alpha	-33,33	-13,04	-5,26	0,00
Beta low frequency	22,22	-3,03	-23,53	21,21
Beta high frequency	25,00	-10,34	-33,33	4,00

When studying lateralization and interhemispheric asymmetry coefficients (IAC) of multiple regression indicators oriented to EEG rhythms within a single lead (i.e., their representation in the left and right hemispheres, Table 4.2), it was found that in right-handers under normal conditions, IAC of delta, theta, low-frequency beta, and high-frequency beta rhythms were oriented to the left hemisphere, while the alpha rhythm was oriented to the right hemisphere.

In left-handers under normal conditions, the IAC of delta, alpha, and both high- and low-frequency beta rhythms were oriented to the right hemisphere, while the theta rhythm was oriented to the left hemisphere. In intellectually disabled right-handers, IAC of all EEG rhythms were oriented to the right hemisphere. In intellectually disabled left-handers, IAC of delta and theta rhythms were oriented to the left hemisphere, while beta rhythms were oriented to the right hemisphere. The IAC of the alpha rhythm was not determined.

Discussion. Multiple regression analysis of amplitude relationships in individuals with intellectual disabilities revealed a greater number of regression coefficients compared to normal conditions, both in left-handers and right-handers. It is noteworthy that under normal conditions, left-handers had more regression coefficients between EEG rhythm amplitudes within a single lead than right-handers.

Similar relationships were found when analyzing amplitude relationships within the same EEG rhythm across different leads [18]. Apparently, the obtained results reflect features of the brain's semantic-topological network.

A greater number of regression coefficients within a single lead was observed in the left hemisphere of right-handers under normal conditions and in the right hemisphere of left-handers. In individuals with intellectual disabilities, the opposite pattern was observed: right-handers had more regression coefficients in the right hemisphere, and left-handers (albeit slightly) in the left hemisphere. An increase in the number of correlations between different EEG and ECoG components reflects an overall increase in cortical tone, while a decrease indicates a reduction in tone.

Therefore, it can be assumed that, according to regression analysis of EEG rhythm amplitude relationships within a single lead, the cortical tone of the left hemisphere is higher than that of the right hemisphere in right-handers under normal conditions. Conversely, in left-handers, the cortical tone of the right hemisphere is higher than that of the left.

In individuals with intellectual disabilities, the cortical tone in right-handers is higher in the right hemisphere than in the left. In left-handers with intellectual disabilities, the cortical tone of the left hemisphere slightly exceeds that of the right.

In different leads, both in left-handers and right-handers with intellectual disabilities, various numbers of relationship connections were determined. These differences may indicate that the activity levels of different brain regions are not uniform. Under normal conditions, in right-handers, higher activity was observed in the C3-P3 (central-parietal) lead in the left hemisphere and the F8-T4 (temporal-central) lead in the right hemisphere. In left-handers, the most active leads were T3-T5 (posterior temporal) in the left hemisphere and T4-T6 (posterior temporal) in the right hemisphere.

Among intellectually disabled right-handers, the greatest number of relationship connections in the left hemisphere was found in the T3-T5 (posterior temporal) lead – 10 connections, and in the right hemisphere in the FP2-F8 (anterior-temporal) lead – 18 connections, indicating these regions are more active than others.

The fewest relationship connections among intellectually disabled right-handers were observed in the T5-O1 (temporal-occipital) lead –4 connections in the left hemisphere, and in the P4-O2 (parietal-occipital) lead –4 connections in the right hemisphere, suggesting these regions are less active than others.

Among intellectually disabled left-handers, the greatest number of relationship connections was found in the C3-P3 (central-parietal) lead in the left hemisphere and the T6-O2 (temporal-occipital) lead in the right hemisphere, indicating these regions are more active than others.

The fewest relationship connections among intellectually disabled left-handers were found in the F7-T3 (temporal-central) lead in the left hemisphere and the C4-P4 (central-parietal) lead in the right hemisphere, suggesting these regions are less active than others.

It can also be hypothesized that the identified connections in the leads reflect projections of EEG rhythm generators into these leads.

The presented findings seemingly support the correctness of considering regression connections, computed through the analysis of relationships between EEG rhythm amplitudes, as units of neurophysiological activity. "With a simple unit, complex phenomena can be described as systematically composed of simple parts. This is the essence of the highly effective strategy known as 'scientific analysis'" (Miller J., Galanter E., Pribram K., 2000).

The analysis of the number of relationship connections oriented to EEG rhythms revealed that both in normal and intellectually disabled right-handers, more connections were oriented to the right hemisphere, while in left-handers, the orientation was less defined.

The presented polycyclic multigraphs, describing amplitude relationships within the same rhythm across different leads, as well as those presented earlier in our work (Lobasyuk B. A., Bartsevich L. B., Zamkovaya A. V., 2022) (Figures 4.5A, 4.5B), illustrate the semantic-topological network model of brain electrical activity.

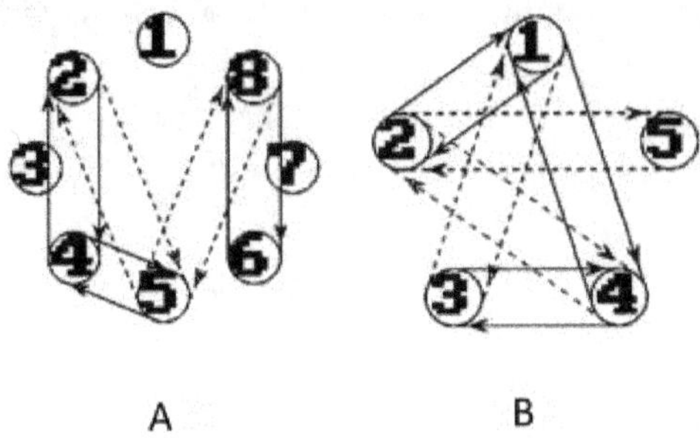

A   B

Figure 4.5. Polycyclic Multigraphs Describing Relationships of Rhythm Amplitude Within the Same Rhythm Across Different Leads (A) and Across Different Rhythms Within the Same Lead (B)

Legend: A: 1 – C3–P3 (Central–Parietal), 2 – F3–C3 (Frontal–Central), 3 – F7–T3 (Temporal–Central), 4 – FP1–F3 (Frontal), 5 – FP1–F7 (Fronto–Temporal), 6 – P3–O1 (Parieto–Occipital), 7 – T3–T5 (Posterior–Temporal), 8 – T5–O1 (Temporo–Occipital).
B: 1 – Delta, 2 – Theta, 3 – Alpha, 4 – Beta (low-frequency), 5 – Beta (high-frequency).

Solid lines indicate positive influences, dashed lines indicate negative influences.

Conclusions:

1. When calculating multiple regression coefficients for EEG rhythm amplitudes in individuals with intellectual disabilities, a greater number of multiple regression coefficients was found. This may be due to the formation of compensatory neurophysiological mechanisms in individuals with intellectual disabilities.

2. When calculating multiple regression coefficients for amplitudes within the same lead in the control group of left-handers, more multiple regression coefficients were found compared to the control group of right-handers. It can be assumed that left-handers have increased cortical tone compared to right-handers.

3. The results presented in points 1 and 2 were also obtained when calculating multiple regression coefficients for EEG rhythm amplitudes within the same frequency range. These findings can be interpreted as a feature of the brain's semantic-topological network organization.

4. In different leads, both in left-handers and right-handers, under normal conditions and in individuals with intellectual disabilities, a varying number of connections (relationships) was determined. The observed differences may indicate that the level of activity in different brain regions is not uniform.

5. A network-based semantic-topological model of brain electrical activity in individuals with intellectual disabilities is described.

Chapter 5.

Network Semantic-Topological Model of Electrogenesis

Understanding the nature and mechanisms of electroencephalogram (EEG) genesis, a method widely used in clinical practice, is highly relevant; however, the mechanisms of EEG generation remain unclear.

In neurophysiology, the concept of multidimensionality of physiological space (its additional dimensions) remains underdeveloped. The hypothesis of multidimensional internal space requires the development of mathematical models in which this phenomenon can be visualized and studied.

The problem of the theory of multilevel systems, known in biomedical interpretations as the "problem of hierarchy in living systems," represents an important stage in the development of general systems theory (Bertalanffy L., 1969). Structure is an integral property of a system, representing a specific type of connection between its elements.

There are various definitions of the concept of "space," making it necessary to clarify the one used in this context. Space is a set of objects between which relationships are established that are structurally similar to conventional spatial relationships, such as neighborhood and distance. Topology deals with solving such problems. The term "topology" first appeared in 1847 in Listing's work: "By topology, we mean the study of modal relations of spatial figures or the laws of connectivity, relative positions, and sequences of points, lines, surfaces, bodies, and their parts or aggregates in space, regardless of measures and magnitudes" (Listing J.B., 1932).

Dynamic functional connections between different areas of the cortex and subcortical structures should play a leading role in brain function, making the problem of intercentral relationships of bio-potentials a key issue (Rusinov V.S., 1987). The formation of functional connections between brain regions can be assessed through the synchronization of their electrical activity (Gasser T., Christine Jennen-Steinmetz Ch., Rolf Verleger R., 1987). For this purpose, the two-dimensional correlation coefficient is calculated. However, this approach cannot determine the directionality of influence since the correlation coefficient $R_{xy} = R_{yx}$. To solve this problem, classical methods of mathematical statistics, such as multiple regression and correlation analysis, can be applied. Using these methods, all identified relationships are oriented, meaning they are directed from one object to another and are direct (not indirect). The systems approach is based on studying the properties of the whole as a whole. A possible solution for the synthesis of objects in multidimensional research is the geometric interpretation of multiple linear regression equations using polycyclic multigraphs—a mathematical language for the formalized representation of concepts related to the analysis and synthesis of structures, systems, and processes—for their subsequent structural analysis.

The aim of this study is to investigate, using multiple linear regression, the relationships between EEG rhythm amplitudes both within a single lead (i.e., between different rhythms) and within a single rhythm between different leads. This approach allows for an integrative assessment of electrogenesis features.

Own Research. Left Hemisphere. A total of 44 regression relationships between EEG rhythm amplitudes within a single lead (i.e., between different rhythms) were identified in the left hemisphere of right-handed individuals (Fig. 1A), while 62 such relationships were found in left-handed individuals (Fig. 5.1B).

Between EEG rhythm amplitudes within a single rhythm across different leads, 36 regression relationships were identified in the left hemisphere of right-handed individuals (Fig. 1B), compared to 42 in left-handed individuals (Fig. 5.1D).

Left Hemisphere, Right-Handed Individuals

Within a single lead, the highest number of regression relationships between different EEG rhythms was found in the central-parietal lead (C3-P3) with 12 relationships, and the lowest was found in the parietal-occipital (P3-O1) and temporal-occipital (T5-O1) leads with 2 relationships each (Fig. 5.1A).

Within a single rhythm across different leads, the highest number of regression relationships was identified in the low-frequency beta rhythm (14 relationships) and the high-frequency alpha and beta rhythms (10 relationships each). The lowest number was found in the delta range (0 relationships) and theta rhythm (2 relationships) (Fig. 5.1B).

Left Hemisphere, Left-Handed Individuals. Within a single lead, the highest number of regression relationships between different EEG rhythms was found in the posterior temporal lead (T3-T5) with 14 relationships, followed by the central-parietal lead (C3-P3) with 12 relationships. The lowest number was found in the frontal lead (FP1-F3) (Fig. 1C).

Left-handers have the highest number of amplitude correlations between different leads within the same rhythm in the left hemisphere.

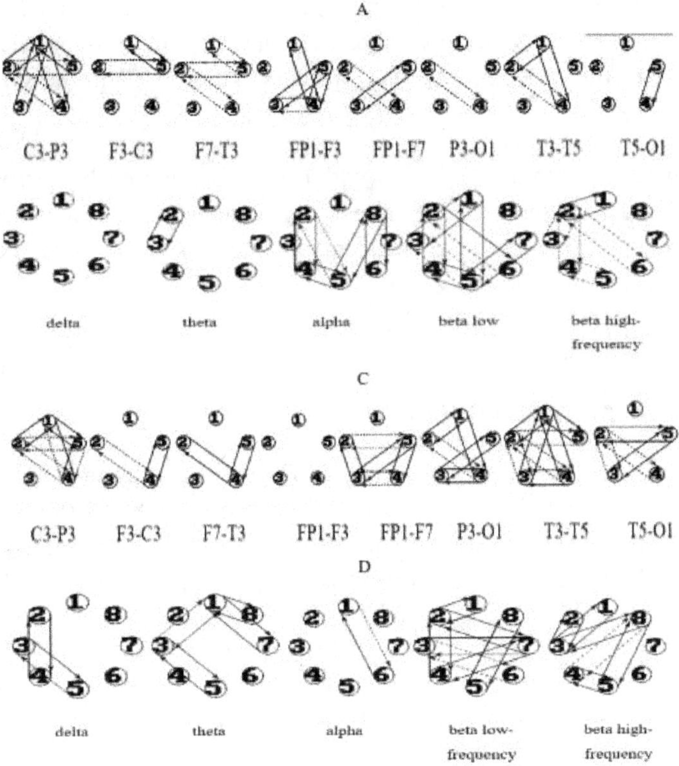

Figure 5.1. Polycyclic Multigraphs Reflecting Relationships Between EEG Rhythm Amplitudes Within a Single Electrode Pair (A, B) and Within a Single Rhythm (C, D) in Right-Handed (A, C) and Left-Handed (B, D) Individuals in the Left Hemisphere

Electrode pairs (A, B): C3–P3 – Central-parietal, F3–C3 – Frontal-central, F7–T3 – Temporal-central, FP1–F3 – Frontal, FP1–F7 – Anterior-temporal, P3–O1 – Parieto-occipital, T3–T5 – Posterior-temporal, T5–O1 – Temporo-occipital, **EEG rhythms (C, D):** Delta, Theta, Alpha, Low-frequency beta, High-frequency beta.

The numbers in the nodes of graphs A and B represent EEG rhythms, while the numbers in the nodes of graphs C and D represent electrode pairs.

Solid lines indicate positive influences, and dashed lines indicate negative influences.

Right Hemisphere

In total, between EEG rhythm amplitudes within a single lead (i.e., between different rhythms), right-handers exhibited 32 regression connections-relations in the right hemisphere (Fig. 5.2, A), while left-handers exhibited 72 in the same situation (Fig. 5.2, B).

Between EEG rhythm amplitudes within a single rhythm but across different leads, right-handers exhibited 22 regression connections-relations in the left hemisphere (Fig. 5.2, C), while left-handers exhibited 44 in the same situation (Fig. 5.2, D).

Right Hemisphere, Right-Handers

Within a single lead, between different EEG rhythms, right-handers exhibited the highest number of regression connections-relations in the F8–T4 (temporal-central) lead (12 connections), and the lowest number in the C4–P4 (central-parietal), FP2–F4 (frontal), and FP2–F8 (anterior-temporal) leads (Fig. 5.2, A).

Within a single rhythm, between amplitudes of different leads, right-handers exhibited the highest number of regression connections-relations in the delta rhythm (14 connections) and the lowest in the low-frequency beta and high-frequency beta rhythms (0 connections) (Fig. 5.2, B).

Right Hemisphere, Left-Handers

Within a single lead, between different EEG rhythms, left-handers exhibited the highest number of regression connections-relations in the T4–T6 (posterior-temporal) lead (18 connections) and the lowest in the FP2–F4 (frontal) lead (Fig. 5.2, C).

Within a single rhythm, between amplitudes of different leads, left-handers exhibited the highest number of regression connections-relations in the low-frequency beta rhythm (18 connections) and the lowest in the theta and high-frequency beta rhythms (4 connections each) (Fig. 5.2, D).

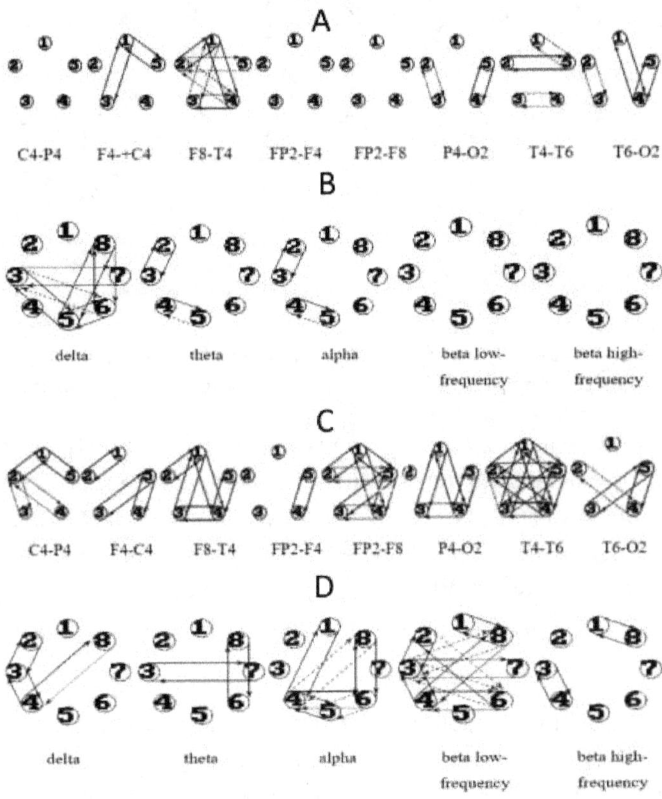

Figure 5.2. Polycyclic Multigraphs Representing Relationships Between EEG Rhythm Amplitudes Within a Single Electrode Pair (A, C) and Within a Single Rhythm (B, D) in Right-Handed (A, B) and Left-Handed (C, D) Individuals in the Right Hemisphere

Electrode Pairs (A, C): 1 — C4–P4 (Central–Parietal), 2 — F4–C4 (Frontal–Central), 3 — F8–T4 (Temporal–Central), 4 — FP2–F4 (Frontal), 5 — FP2–F8 (Anterior–Temporal), 6 — P4–O2 (Parietal–Occipital), 7 — T4–T6 (Posterior–Temporal), 8 — T6–O2 (Temporal–Occipital),

EEG Rhythms (B, D): 1 — Delta, 2 — Theta, 3 — Alpha, 4 — Low-Frequency Beta, 5 — High-Frequency Beta

The numbers in the graph nodes represent: **In graphs A and B:** EEG rhythms, **In graphs C and D:** Electrode pairs

75

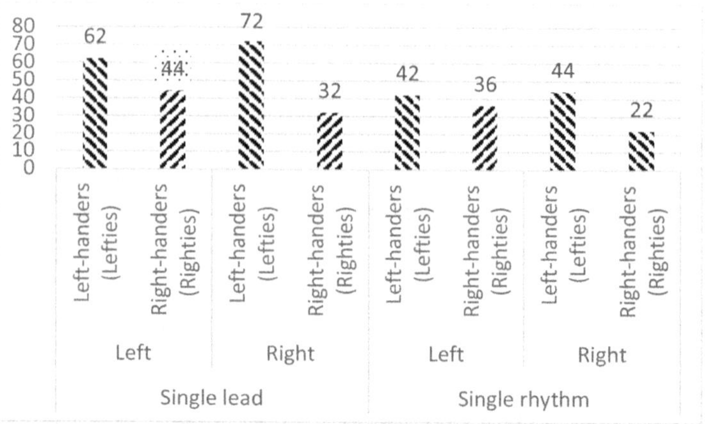

Figure 5.3. The Number of Regression Links-Relations Within a Single Electrode and Rhythm. Designations: left – left hemisphere, right – right hemisphere

Discussion. When calculating regression coefficients between EEG rhythm amplitudes within a single rhythm, left-handers showed 1.16 times more regression coefficients in the left hemisphere and twice as many in the right hemisphere. When calculating regression coefficients between EEG rhythm amplitudes within a single electrode but across different EEG rhythms, left-handers showed 1.4 times more regression coefficients in the left hemisphere and 2.25 times more in the right hemisphere.

Thus, both within a single EEG rhythm and within a single electrode across different rhythms, left-handers exhibited more regression coefficients between EEG rhythm amplitudes than right-handers. It can be assumed that left-handers have an increased cortical tone compared to right-handers.

In both left-handers and right-handers, the greatest number of links-relations within a single electrode in the left hemisphere was found in the central-parietal lead C3–P3. It can be assumed that this lead is a kind of focus for the influence of various EEG rhythm generators in the left hemisphere. Among right-handers, the greatest number of links-relations within a single electrode in the right hemisphere was found in the temporal-central lead F8–T4, while among left-handers, it was in the posterior-temporal lead T4–T6. It can be assumed that these leads serve as focal points for the influence of various EEG rhythm generators in the right hemisphere.

When calculating the number of regression coefficients for right-handers within a single rhythm between different electrodes, the highest number of coefficients in the left hemisphere was found in the low-frequency beta (beta-LF), high-frequency beta (beta-HF), and alpha rhythms, with the lowest in delta and theta rhythms. In the right hemisphere, the opposite pattern was observed—the highest number of regression coefficients was in the delta rhythm and the lowest in beta-LF and beta-HF rhythms.

When calculating the number of regression coefficients for left-handers within a single rhythm between different electrodes, the highest number of links-relations in the left hemisphere, similar to right-handers, was found in the beta-LF and beta-HF rhythms, and the lowest in the alpha rhythm. In the right hemisphere, the highest number of links-relations was found in the beta-LF rhythm, and the lowest in the theta and beta-HF rhythms.

The results suggest that beta-LF and beta-HF rhythms act as the primary integrative rhythms of electrogenesis for right-handers in the left hemisphere and for left-handers in both hemispheres. For right-handers, the delta rhythm appears to be the primary integrative rhythm in the right hemisphere.

Based on the above, it can be assumed that the structure of the electrogenesis system is reticular and has topological properties.

Previously, we developed a concept of the unit of mental activity as a psycho-psychiatric and neurophysiological construct based on multiple regression analysis of EEG indicators and the anxiety index from the Luscher test (Bitensky, V.S., Lobasyuk, B.A., Bodelan, M.I., 2010). Considering the results obtained in this study, the unit of neurophysiological activity can be represented as a regression link-relation between EEG indicators.

Thus, the mathematical model of electrogenesis obtained by us allows it to be classified as a labile reticular-topological structure.

Conclusions:

1. Left-handers exhibit a greater number of regression coefficients between EEG rhythm amplitudes than right-handers. This may indicate increased cortical tone in left-handers compared to right-handers.
2. The central-parietal lead C3–P3 serves as a focal point of influence from various EEG rhythm generators in the left hemisphere.

3. Beta-LF and beta-HF rhythms are the primary integrative rhythms of electrogenesis for right-handers in the left hemisphere and for left-handers in both hemispheres. The delta rhythm is the primary integrative rhythm in the right hemisphere for right-handers.
4. The mathematical model of brain electrogenesis obtained in this study allows it to be classified as a labile reticular-topological structure.

Literature

1. Листинг И.Б. Предварительные исследования по топологии. (Vorstudien zur topologie, 1848). Перевод с немецкого под редакцией и с предисловием Э.Кольмана. (Москва - Ленинград: Гостехиздат, 1932. - Классики естествознания). 156 с.

2. Лобасюк Б.А. Системные нейрофизиологические механизмы электрогенеза головного мозга. ХГЭУ. Одесса. 2010. 424 с.

3. Лобасюк Б.А., Боделан М.И. Взаимоотношения ритмов ЭЭГ разных отведений. // The unity of science. N 4. Vienna, Austria, 2016.

4. Мангейм Дж. Б., Рич Р. К. Политология. Методы исследования, Весь Мир, Москва (1997

5. Миллер Дж., Галантер Е., Прибрам К. Программы и стоуктура повежения. Методические рекомендации для слушателей курса "НЛП в бизнесе". Москва, 2000 - 228 стр. ISBN 5-7856-0196-6

6. Abou Elseoud, Ahmed; Littow, Harri; Remes, Jukka; Starck, Tuomo; Nikkinen, Juha; Nissilä, Juuso; Timonen, Markku; Tervonen, Osmo; Kiviniemi1, Vesa (2011-06-03). "Group-ICA Model Order Highlights Patterns of Functional Brain Connectivity". Frontiers in Systems Neuroscience. 5:37. doi:10.3389/fnsys.2011.00037. PMC 3109774. PMID 2 1687724.

7. Albada van S.J., Robinson P.A. Relationships between Electroencephalographic Spectral Peaks Across Frequency Bands. Front Hum Neurosci. 2013 4; 7:56.

8. Albada van S.J., Robinson P.A. Relationships between Electroencephalographic Spectral Peaks Across Frequency Bands. Front Hum Neurosci. 2013 4; 7:56.

9. Andersen P. A. Andersson S. A. Holmgren E. Theoretical consideration on the synchronization of thalamo-cortical activity Subcortical Mechanisms and Sensorimotor Activities / Ed. Frigyesi Bern: Huber. 1975. – P. 229-250.

10. Andrews-Hanna J.R., Smallwood J.N, Spreng R. N. The default network and self-generated thought: component processes, dynamic control, and clinical relevance // Annals of the New York

11. Bailey, S. K.; Aboud, K.S.; Nguyen, T. Q.; C., Laurie E. (13 December 2018). "Applying a network framework to the neurobiology of reading and dyslexia". Journal of Neurodevelopmental Disorders. 10 (1): 37.

doi:10.1186/s11689-018-9251-z. PMC 6291929. PMID 30541433.

12. Bak P, Tang C, Wiesenfeld K. Self-organized criticality: an explanation of the 1/f noise. Phys Rev Lett 1987;27(59):381–4.

13. Barrat A, Barthelemy M, Vespignami A. Dynamical processes on complex networks. Cambridge: Cambridge University Press; 2008

14. Basar E. Brain function and oscillations. – Berlin. New York: Springer. 1998. – 467 p.

15. Basar E., Shurmann M. Alpha rhythms in the brain: functional correlates // News. Physiol. Sci. 1996. V. 11. P. 90–96.

16. Basar E., Shurmann M. Alpha rhythms in the brain: functional correlates // Ns. Physiol. Sci. 1996. V. 11. P. 90–96.

17. Beggs J.M., Plenz D. Neuronal avalanches in neocortical circuits. J Neurosci 2003; 23:11167–77.

18. Bell, Peter T.; Shine, James M. (2015-11-09). "Estimating Large-Scale Network Convergence in the Human Functional Connectome". Brain Connectivity. 5 (9):565–74. doi:10.1089/brain.2015.0348. PMID 26005099.

19. Bertalanffy Ludwig von The Theory of Open Systems in Physics and Biology// Science 13 January 1950 111: 23-29 [DOI: 10.1126/science.111.2872.23] (in Articles)

20. Besthorn C., Förstl H., Geiger C.-KabischH.SattelT.GasserU.Schreiter-Gasser EEG coherence in Alzheimer disease. Electroencephalography and Clinical Neurophysiology Volume 90, Issue 3, March 1994, Pages 242-245 https://doi.org/10.1016/0013-4694(94)90095-7

21. Boccaletti S, Kurths J, Osipov G, Valladares DL, Zhou CS. The synchronization of chaotic systems. Phys Rep 2002; 366:1–101.

22. Boccaletti S, Kurths J, Osipov G, Valladares DL, Zhou CS. The synchronization of chaotic systems. Phys Rep 2002; 366:1–101.

23. Boccaletti S, Latora V, Moreno Y, Chavez M, Hwang D-U. Complex networks: structure and dynamics. Phys Rep 2006; 424:175–308.

24. Boccaletti S, Latora V, Moreno Y, Chavez M, Hwang D-U. Complex networks: structure and dynamics. Phys Rep 2006; 424:175–308.

25. Bressler, S. L.; Menon, V. (June 2010). "Large scale brain networks in cognition: emerging methods and rprinciples". Trends in Cognitive Sciences. 14 (6): 233–290.
doi:10.1016/j.tics.2010.04.004. PMID 20493761. S2CID 5967761.
Retrieved 24 January 2016.

26. Bressler, S.L. (2008). "Neurocognitive networks". Scholarpedia. 3 (2): 1567. Bibcode:2008SchpJ...3.1567B. doi:10.4249/scholarpedia.1567.

27. Bressler, Steven L.; Menon, Vinod (June 2010). "Large scale brain networks in cognition: emerging methods and principles". Trends in Cognitive Sciences. 14 (6): 233–290. doi:10.1016/j.tics.2010.04.004. PMID 20493761. S2CID 5967761. Retrieved 24 January 2016.

28. Buckner, Randy L. (2012-08-15). "The serendipitous discovery of the brain's default network". NeuroImage. 62 (2): 1137–1145. doi:10.1016/j.neuroimage.2011.10.035. ISSN 1053-119. PMID 22037421. S2CID 9880586.

29. Buckner, R.L., Hanna A., Daniel L. S. The Brain's Default Network Anatomy, Function, and Relevance to Disease. https://doi.org/10.1196/annals.1440.011

30. Bullmore E., Sporns O. The economy of brain network organization- Nature Reviews Neuroscience, 2012-13 (5): 336-349, http: // dx.doi.org/10.1038/nrn3214.

31. Carracedo L.M., Kjeldsen H., Cunnington L., Jenkins A., Schofield I., Cunningham M.O., Davies C.H., Traub R.D., Whittington M.A. A neocortical delta rhythm facilitates reciprocal interlaminar interactions via nested theta rhythms.J Neurosci. 2013 Jun 26;33(26):10750-61.

32. Cohn R. The occipital alpha rhythm: a study of phase variations / Cohn R. // J.Neurophysiol. – 1948. – V. 11. – P. 31–37.

33. Dubois B. 0[etal м. The 0FAB: ам frontal assessmentbatter yatbedside.Neurology, 2000,vol. 55, no. 3, pp. 1621-1626.

34. Eickhoff, S.B.; Yeo, B.T.T., Genon, S., (November 2018). "Imaging-based parcellations of the human brain"(PDF). Nature Reviews. Neuroscience.19 (11): 672–686.doi:10.1038/s41583-018-0071-7.PMID. S2CID 52954265.

35. ElbleR.J. Characteristicof physiologic tremorinyo ungandelderlyadults. J.Clin Neurophysiol, 2003, no.114, suppl. 4, no.624-635.

36. Flor-Henry, P., Koles Z. J. (1982). EEG characteristics of normal subjects: A comparison of men and women and of dextrals and sinistrals. Research Communications in Psychology, Psychiatry & Behavior, 7(1), 21–38.

37. Foster, Brett L.; Parvizi, Josef (2012-03-01). "Resting oscillations and cross-frequency coupling in the human posteromedial cortex". NeuroImage. 60 (1): 384–391. doi:10.1016/j.neuroimage.2011.12.019. ISSN 10538119. PMC 3596417. P MID 22227048.

38. Frontiers in Psychology. 3: 295. doi:10.3389/fpsyg.2012.00295. PMC 3427917.PMID 22969735.

39. Gasser T., Christine Jennen-Steinmetz Ch., Rolf Verleger R., EEG coherence at rest and during a visual task in two groups of children Electroencephalography and Clinical Neurophysiology. Volume 67, Issue 2, 1987, P. 151-158.

40. Griffiths, Kristi R.; Braund, Taylor A.; Kohn, Michael R.; Clarke, Simon; Williams, Leanne M.; Korgaonkar, Mayuresh S. (2 March 2021). "Structural brain network topology underpinning ADHD and response to methylphenidate treatment". Translational Psychiatry. 11 (1): 150. doi:10.1038/s41398-021-01278-x. PMC 7925571. PMID 33654073.

41. Growdon W., Ghika J., Henderson J. Effects of proximal and distalmuscles' groups' contraction and mental stress on the amplitude and frequency of physiological finger tremor. Anaccelerometric study. Electromyogr Clin Neurophysiol, 2000, no.40, suppl. 5, pp.295-303.

42. Gurfinkel' V. S., KotsYa. M., Shik M. L. Regulyatsiya pozy cheloveka [Regulation of human posture]. Moscow, Science Publ., 1965, 256 p. (In Russ.)

43. Hallett M. Over view of human tremor physiology. Movement Disorders, 1998, no. 13, suppl. 3, 43-48.

44. Hutton, John S.; Dudley, Jonathan; Horowitz-Kraus, Tzipi; DeWitt, Tom; Holland, Scott K. (1 September 2019)."Functional Connectivity of Attention, Visual, and Language Networks During Audio, Illustrated, and Animated Stories in Preschool-Age Children". Brain Connectivity. 9 (7): 580–592. doi:10.1089/brain.2019.0679. PMC 6775495. PMID 31144523.

45. Buckner R.L., Andrews-Hanna J.R., Schacter D.L. The brain's default network: anatomy, function, and relevance to disease. Annals of the new York Academy of Sciences, 2008•Wiley Online Libra

46. Bassett, Daniella; Bertolero, Max (July 2019). "How Matter Becomes Mind". Scientific American. 321 (1): 32. Retrieved 23 June 2019.

47. Heine, Lizette; Soddu, Andrea; Gomez, Francisco; Vanhaudenhuyse, Audrey; Tshibanda, Luaba; Thonnard, Marie; Charland-Verville, Vanessa; Kirsch, Murielle; Laureys, Steven; Demertzi, Athena (2012)."Resting state networks and consciousness. Alterations of multiple resting state network connectivity in physiological, pharmacological and pathological consciousness sta

48. Kanda P.A.M., Anghinah R., Magali Taino Smidth M.T., Jorge Mario Silva J.M. The clinical use of quantitative EEG in cognitive disorders A utilizaçãoclínica do EEG quantitativo nos transtornos cognitivos. Dement. neuropsychol. 3 (3) 2009.

https://doi.org/10.1590/S1980-57642009DN30300004.

49. Khazi M., Kumar A., Dept V.M. Analysis of EEG Using 10:20 Electrode System. International Journal of Innovative Research in Science, Engineering and Technology Vol. 1, Issue 2, 2012.

50. Korenkevych D, Chien J.H,, Zhang J. Small world networks in computational neuroscience. Handbook of, 2013 - jhu.pure.elsevier.com

51. Korenkevych D., Chien J.-H, Zhang J., Deng Shan Shiau D,-C,, Chris Sackellares Ch., Pardalos P.M.

52. L. Von Bertalanffy, "General theory of system application to psychology," Soc. Sci. Inform. Sci. Soc., No. 6, 126-136 (1967).

53. Lehmann, D. Human scalp EEG fields:evoked, alpha, sleep and spike-wave patterns / D. Lehmann // Synchronization of EEG Activity in Epilepsies. – New York: Springer-Verlag, 1972. – P. 307-326.

54. Lobasyuk B. A., Bartsevich L. B., Zamkovaya A. V. Application of multiple regression analysis to study the relationship between eeg rhythms at persons with mental retardation. Journal f Education, Health and Sport. 2022;12(2):232-248. Eissn

55. Lobasyuk B.A., Bartsevich L.B., Zamkovaya A.V. Application of multiple regression analysis to study the relationship between eeg rhythms кат persons with mental retardation. Journal of Education, Health and Sport. 2022; 12(2):232-248. eISSN 2391-8306. DOI http://dx.doi.org/10.12775/JEHS.2022.12.02.025

56. Lobasyuk B.A. Role of the brainstem reticular formation in the mechanisms of cortical electrogenesis. 2005.- Neurophysiology -V. 37, №1. – C.39-45.

57. Locatellia T., M.Cursia M., D.Liberatib D.,, M.Franceschia M., Comia G. EEG coherence in Alzheimer's disease Electroencephalography and Clinical Neurophysiology. Volume 106, Issue 3, March 1998, Pages 229-237

58. Lopes da Silva F.H. van Lierop T.H.M.T. Schrijer C.F.M. Storm van Leeuwen W. Essential differences between alpha rhythm and barbiturate spindles: spectra and thalamo-cortical coherence Electroenceph. clin. – 1973b. – V. 35. – P. 626-639.

59. Mangeym B., Rich P.K., Politologiya. Metodyi issledovaniya, Ves Mir, Moskva (1997).

60. Marco-Pallarés J., Grau C., Location of brain rhythms and their modulation by preparatory attention estimated by current density C.M.Gómez[a] Brain Research Volume 1107, Issue 1, 30 August 2006, Pages 151-160.

61. Marek, Scott; Dosenbach, Nico U. F. (June 2018). "The frontoparietal network: function, electrophysiology, and importance of individual precision mapping". Dialogues in Clinical Neuroscience. 20 (2):133–140. doi:10.31887/DCNS.2018.20.2/smarek.ISSNm1294-8322. PMC 6136121. PMID 30250390.

62. McAuleyJ.H., MarsdenC.D. Physiological and pathological tremor sandrhythmic central motor control. Brain, 2000, no. 123, suppl. 8, pp.1545-1567.

63. Menon, V. (2015-01-01), "Salience Network", in Toga, Arthur W. (ed.), Brain Mapping, Academic Press, pp. 597–611, doi:10.1016/B978-0-12-397025-1.00052-X, ISBN 978-0-12-397316-0, retrieved 2019-12-08

64. Menon, Vinod (2011-09-09)."Large-scale brain networks and psychopathology: A unifying triple network model".Trends in Cognitive Sciences. 15 (10): 483–506. doi:10.1016/j.tics.2011.08.003. PMID 21908230. S2CID 26653572.

65. Michael D.; Corbetta, Maurizio; Snyder, Abraham Z.; Vincent, Justin L.; Raichle, Marcus E. (2006-06-27). "Spontaneous neuronal activity distinguishes human dorsal and ventral attention systems". Proceedings of the National Academy of Sciences.103 (26): 10046–10051. Bibcode:2006PNAS..10310046F.doi:10.1073/pnas.0604187103. ISSN 0027-8424. PMC 1480402. PMID 16788060.

66. Michel C.M., Lehmann D., Henggeler B., Brandeis D. Localization of the sources of EEG delta, theta, alpha and beta frequency bands using the FFT dipole approximation.//Electroencephalogr Clin Neurophysiol. 1992; 82(1):38-44.

67. Michel C.M., Lehmann D., Henggeler B., Brandeis D. Localization of the sources of EEG delta, theta, alpha and beta frequency bands using the FFT dipole approximation.//Electroencephalogr Clin Neurophysiol. 1992; 82(1):38-44.

68. Morris, Peter G.; Smith, Stephen M.; Barnes, Gareth R.; Stephenson, Mary C.; Hale, Joanne R.; Price, Darren; Luckhoo, Henry; Woolrich, Mark; Brookes, Matthew J. (2011-10-04)."Investigating the electrophysiological basis of resting state networks using magnetoencephalography". Proceedings of the National Academy of Sciences. 108 (40): 16783–16788.Bibcode:2011PNAS..10816783B.doi:10.1073/pnas.1112685108. ISS N 0027-8424.PMC 3189080. PMID 21930901.

69. n S.A. Thalamic origin of cortical rhythmic activity / Handbook of Electroencephalography and Clinical Neurophysiology / Ed. Amsterdam: Elsevier. 1974. – Vol. 2, – P. 90

70. Network". Annals of the New York Academy of Sciences. 1124 (1): 1–38. Bibcode:2008NYASA1124....1B. doi:10.1196/annals.1440.011. ISSN 1 749-6632. PMID 18400922. S2CID 3167595.

71. Nunez PL. Brain, mind, and the structure of reality. Oxford University Press; 2010.

72. O'Suilleabhain P.E., Matsumoto J.Y. Time-frequency analysis of tremors. Brain, 1998, no. 121, pp. 2127-2124.

73. Pardalos B: Du P.M, Graham D.-Z., RL (editors). Combinatorial Optimization Reference. New York: Springer; 2013; p. 3057-3088

74. Petersen, Steven; Sporns, Olaf (October 2015)."Brain Networks and Cognitive Architectures". Neuron. 88 (1): 207–219. doi:10.1016/j.neuron.2015.09.027. PMC 4598639. PMID 26447582.

75. Petersen, Steven; Sporns, Olaf (October 2015). "Brain Networks and Cognitive Architectures". Neuron. 88 (1): 207–219. doi:10.1016/j.neuron.2015.09.027. PMC 4598639. PMID 26447582.

76. Raethjen J., Pawlas F., Lindemann M. [et al.] Determinants of physiologic tremor in a large normal population. J.ClinNeurophysiol, 2000,no. 111, suppl. 10, pp. 1825-1837

77. Raichle Marcus E. The Brain's Default Mode Network // Annual Review of Neuroscience. — 2015. — Vol. 38. — P. 433-447. — ISSN 0147-006X. — doi:10.1146/annurev-neuro-071013-014030

78. Raichle Marcus E. The Brain's Default Mode Network // Annual Review of Neuroscience. — 2015.— Vol.38.— P.433-447.—ISSN 0147-006X.— doi:10.1146/annurev-neuro-071013-014030

79. Riedl V.; Utz L.; Castrillón G. et sll. 2016; Bressler Steven L.; Menon, V. 2010; Yeo, B. T. Thomas; Krienen, Fenna M.; Sepulcre J. 2011).

80. Riedl V., Utz L. C., Gabriel G., Timo R, J. P.; Ploner M.F., Friston, K.J.; Drzezga A., Sorg Ch. (January 12, 2016)."Metabolic connectivity mapping reveals effective connectivity in the resting human brain".PNAS.113(2): 428–433.Bibcode:2016PNAS..113..428R. doi:10.1073/pnas.1513752113. PMC 4720331. PMID 26712010.

81. Riedl, Valentin; Utz, Lukas; Castrillón, Gabriel; Grimmer, Timo; Rauschecker, Josef P.; Ploner, Markus; Friston, Karl J.; Drzezga, Alexander; Sorg, Christian (January 12, 2016). "Metabolic connectivity mapping reveals effective connectivity in the resting human brain". PNAS. 113 (2): 428–

433. Bibcode:2016PNAS..113..428R. doi:10.1073/pnas.1513752113. PMC 4720331. PMID 26712010.

82. Riedl, Valentin; Utz, Lukas; Castrillón, Gabriel; Grimmer, Timo; Rauschecker, Josef P.; Ploner, Markus; Friston, Karl J.; Drzezga, Alexander; Sorg, Christian (January 12, 2016). "Metabolic connectivity mapping reveals effective connectivity in the resting human brain". PNAS. 113 (2): 428–433. Bibcode:2016PNAS..113..428R. doi:10.1073/pnas.1513752113. PMC 4720331. PMID 26712010.

83. S. J. Williamson, L. Kaufman, Z.-L. Lu, et al., "Study of human occipital alpha rhythm: the alphon hypothesis and alpha suppression," Int. J. Psychophysiol., 26(1-3), 63-76 (1997).

84. S.A. Isaychev, D.S. Osipova, Yu.M. Koptelov. Dipolnyie modeli generatora alfa-ritma. Fiziol. Vyissh. Nervnoy (psihicheskoy) deyatelnosti. 2003. T.53. #5. s. 577-586.

85. Scolari, Miranda; Seidl-Rathkopf, Katharina N; Kastner, Sabine (2015-02-01). "Functions of the human frontoparietal attention network: Evidence from neuroimaging". Current Opinion in Behavioral Sciences. Cognitive control. 1:32-39.
doi:10.1016/j.cobeha.2014.08.003. ISSN 23521546. PMC 4936532. PMID 27398396.

86. Shafiei, Golia; Zeighami, Yashar; Clark, Crystal A.; Coull, Jennifer T.; Nagano-Saito, Atsuko; Leyton, Marco; Dagher, Alain; Mišić, Bratislav (2018-10-01). "Dopamine Signaling Modulates the Stability and Integration of Intrinsic Brain Networks". Cerebral Cortex. 29 (1): 397–409. doi:10.1093/cercor/bhy264. PMC 6294404. PMID 30357316.

87. Shannon CE, Weaver W. The mathematical theory of communication. Urbana and Chicago: University of Illinois Press; 1949.

88. Shaw J.C., O'Connor K.P., Ongley C. The EEG as a measure of cerebral functional organization.- The British Journal of Psychiatry, 1977 – 130 (3): 260-264)

89. Shulman, Gordon L.; McAvoy, Mark P.; Cowan, Melanie C.; Astafiev, Serguei V.; Tansy, Aaron P.; d'Avossa, Giovanni; Corbetta, Maurizio (2003-11-01). "Quantitative Analysis of Attention and Detection Signals During Visual Search". Journal of Neurophysiology. 90 (5): 3384–3397. doi:10.1152/jn.00343.2003. ISSN 0022-3077. PMID 12917383.

90. Simon HA. The architecture of complexity. Proc Natl Acad Sci USA 1962; 106:467–82. Simpson Small world networks in computational neuroscience

91. Small world networks in computational neuroscience B: Pardalos P.M, Du D.-Z., Graham RL (editors). Combinatorial Optimization Reference. New York: Springer; 2013; p. 3057-3088

92. Smith, S.M.; Fox, P.T.; Miller, K.L. et al) .10-15). "Evaluation of the spatial variability in the major resting-state networks across human brain functional atlases". Human Brain Mapping. 40 (15): 4577–4587. doi:10.1002/hbm.24722. PMC 6771873. PMID 31322303.

93. Smith, SM; Fox, PT; Miller, KL; Glahn, DC; Fox, PM; Mackay, CE; Filippini, N; Watkins, KE; Toro, R; Laird, AR; Beckmann, CF (2009-08-04). "Correspondence of the brain's functional architecture during activation and rest". Proceedings of the National Academy of Sciences of the United States of America. 106 (31): 13040–5. Bibcode:2009PNAS..10613040S. doi:10.1073/pnas.0905267106. PMC 272 2273. PMID 19620724.

94. Smith, SM; Fox, PT; Miller, KL; Glahn, DC; Fox, PM; Mackay, CE; Filippini, N; Watkins, KE; Toro, R; Laird, AR; Beckmann, CF (2009-08-04). "Correspondence of the brain's functional architecture during activation and rest". Proceedings of the National Academy of Sciences of the United States of America. 106 (31): 13040

95. Bibcode:2009PNAS..10613040S. doi:10.1073/pnas.0905267106. PMC 272 2273. PMID 19620724.

96. Sporns O, Tononi G, Edelman GM. Theoretical neuroanatomy: relating anatomical and functional connectivity in graphs and cortical connection matrices. Cereb Cortex 2000; 10:127–41. Sporns O, Kötter R. Motifs in brain networks. PLoS Biol 2004; 2:e369.

97. Sporns O. Complex network measures of brain connectivity: uses and interpretations. Neuroimage 2010; 52:1059–69.

98. Sporns O. Networks of the brain. Cambridge, Massachusetts: The MIT Press; 2011a.

99. Sporns O. The human connectome: a complex network. Ann NY Acad Sci 2011b;1224: 109–25.

100. Stam CJ. Nonlinear dynamical analysis of EEG and MEG: review of an emerging field. Clin Neurophysiol 2005; 116:2266–301.

101. Stam, E.C.W. van Straaten / Clinical Neurophysiology xxx (2012) xxx–xxx Please cite this article in press as: Stam CJ, van Straaten ECW. The organization of physiological brain networks. Clin Neurophysiol (2012), doi:10.1016/ j.clinph.2012.01.011

102. Steimke, Rosa; Nomi, Jason S.; Calhoun, Vince D.; Stelzel, Christine; Paschke, Lena M.; Gaschler, Robert; Goschke, Thomas; Walter, Henrik; Uddin, Lucina Q. (2017-12-01). "Salience network dynamics underlying successful resistance of temptation". Social Cognitive and Affective Neuroscience. 12 (12): 1928–1939. doi:10.1093/scan/nsx123. ISSN 1749-5016. PMC 5716209. PMID 29048582.

103. Thomas B. T; Krienen, Fenna M.; Sepulcre, Jorge; Sabuncu, Mert R.; Lashkari Danial; Hollinshead, Marisa; Roffman, Joshua L.; Smoller, Jordan W.; Zöllei, Lilla; Polimeni, Jonathan R.; Fischl, Bruce; Liu, Hesheng; Buckner, Randy L. (2011, -09-01). "The organization of the human cerebral cortex estimated by intrinsic functional connectivity". Journal of Neurophysiology. 106 (3): 1125–1165. Bibcode:2011NatSD...2E0031H. doi:10.1152/jn.00338.2011. PMC 3174820. PMID 21653723.

104. Tucker M., Stenslie C.E., Randy S. Roth R.S., MS; Steve L. Shearer S.l. Right Frontal Lobe Activation and Right Hemisphere PerformanceDecrement During a Depressed Mood Arch Gen Psychiatry. 1981;38(2):169-174. doi:10.1001/archpsyc.1981.01780270055007

105. Uddin, L.Q.; Yes, BTT; Spreng, R.N. (November 2019). "Towards a universal taxonomy of macroscale functional networks in the human brain". Topography of the brain. 32(6): 926–942. doi:10.1007/s10548-019-6. PMC 7325607. PMID31707621

106. Uddin, LQ; Yeo, BTT; Spreng, RN (November 2019). "Towards a Universal Taxonomy of Macro-scale Functional Human Brain Networks". Brain Topography. 32 (6): 926–942. doi:10.1007/s10548-019-00744-6. PMC 7325607. PMID 31707621.

107. Uddin, LQ; Yeo, BTT; Spreng, RN (November 2019). "Towards a Universal Taxonomy of Macro-scale Functional Human Brain Networks". Brain Topography. 32 (6): 926–942. doi:10.1007/s10548-019-00744-6. PMC 7325607. PMID 31707621.

108. Uddin, Lucina (10 October 2022). "The Brain Network by Any Other Name". Journal of Cognitive Neuroscience. 2022 (10): 363–364. doi:10.1162/jocn_a_01925. PMID 36223250. S2CID 252844955

109. Uddin, Lucina (2022-10-10). "A Brain Network by Any Other Name". Journal of Cognitive Neuroscience. 2022 (10): 363–364. doi:10.1162/jocn_a_01925. PMID 36223250. S2CID 25284495

110. Uddin, Lucina (2022-10-10). "A Brain Network by Any Other Name". Journal of Cognitive Neuroscience. 2022 (10): 363–364. doi:10.1162/jocn_a_01925. PMID 36223250. S2CID 252844955.

111. von Bertalanffy L. General system theory. Foundations, development, applications. New York: George Braziller

112. Vossel, Simone; Geng, Joy J.; Fink, Gereon R. (2014). "Dorsal and Ventral Attention Systems: Distinct Neural Circuits but Collaborative Roles". The Neuroscientist. 20 (2): 150–159. doi:10.1177/1073858413494269. PMC 4107817. PMID 23835449.

113. Weiss S., Rappelsberger P. Left Frontal EEG Coherence Reflects Modality Independent Language Processes // Brain Topograpy. 1998. Vol. 11. № 1. P. 33–42

114. Weiss S., Rappelsberger P. Left Frontal EEG Coherence Reflects Modality Independent Language Processes // Brain Topograpy. 1998. Vol. 11. № 1. P. 33–42

115. Weiss S., Rappelsberger P. Left Frontal EEG Coherence Reflects Modality Independent Language Processes // Brain Topograpy 1998. Vol. 11. № 1. P. 33–42ith

116. Wiener N. Cybernetics: or control and communication in the animal and the machine. Cambridge, Massachusetts: The MIT Press; 1948.

117. Williamson S. J., Kaufman L., Lu Z.-L., et al., tudy of human occipital alpha rhythm: the alphon hypothesis and alpha suppression,Int. J. Psychophysiol., 26(1-3), 63-76 (1997)

118. Yang, Yan-li; Deng, Hong-xia; Xing, Gui-yang; Xia, Xiao-luan; Li, Hai-fang (2015). "Brain functional network connectivity based on a visual task: visual information processing-related brain regions are significantly activated in the task state". Neural Regeneration Research. 10 (2): 298–307. doi:10.4103/1673-5374.152386. PMC 4392680. PMID 25883631.

119. Yeo, B. T. Thomas; Krienen, Fenna M.; Sepulcre, Jorge; Sabuncu, Mert R.; Lashkari, Danial; Hollinshead, Marisa; Roffman, Joshua L.; Smoller, ordan W.; Zöllei, Lilla; Polimeni, Jonathan R.; Fischl, Bruce; Liu, Hesheng; Buckner, Randy L. (2011-09-01). "The organization of the human cerebral cortex estimated by intrinsic functional connectivity". Journal of Neurophysiology. 106 (3): 1125–1165. Bibcode:2011NatSD...2E0031H. doi:10.1152/jn.00338.2011. PMC 3174820. PMID 21653723.

120. Yuan, Rui; Di, Xin; Taylor, Paul A.; Gohel, Suril; Tsai, Yuan-Hsiung; Biswal, Bharat B. (30 April 2015). "Functional topography of the

thalamocortical system in human". Brain Structure and Function. **221** (4): 1971–1984. doi:10.1007/s00429-015-1018-

7. PMC 6363530. PMID 25924563.

121. Zheng-yan Jiang Study on EEG power and coherence in patients with mild cognitive impairment during working memory task. Journal of Zhejiang University SCIENCE

Literature

1. Listing I.B. Predvaritelnye issledovaniya po topologii. (Vorstudien zur topologie, 1848). Perevod s nemeckogo pod redakciej i s predisloviem E.Kolmana. (Moskva - Leningrad: Gostehizdat, 1932. - Klassiki estestvoznaniya). 156 s.

2. Lobasyuk B.A. Sistemnye nejrofiziologicheskie mehanizmy elektrogeneza golovnogo mozga. HGEU. Odessa. 2010. 424 s.

3. Lobasyuk B.A., Bodelan M.I. Vzaimootnosheniya ritmov EEG raznyh otvedenij. // The unity of science. N 4. Vienna, Austria, 2016.

4. Mangejm, Dzh. B., Rich P. K. Politologiya. Metody issledovaniya, Ves Mir, Moskva (1997

5. Miller Dzh., Galanter E., Pribram K. Programmy i stouktura povezheniya. Metodicheskie rekomendacii dlya slushatelej kursa "NLP v biznese". Moskva, 2000 - 228 str. ISBN 5-7856-0196-6

6. Abou Elseoud, Ahmed; Littow, Harri; Remes, Jukka; Starck, Tuomo; Nikkinen, Juha; Nissila, Juuso; Timonen, Markku; Tervonen, Osmo; Kiviniemi1, Vesa (2011-06-03). "Group-ICA Model Order Highlights Patterns of Functional Brain Connectivity". Frontiers in Systems Neuroscience. 5:37. doi:10.3389/fnsys.2011.00037. PMC 3109774. PMID 21687724.

7. Albada van S.J., Robinson P.A. Relationships between Electroencephalographic Spectral Peaks Across Frequency Bands. Front Hum Neurosci. 2013 4; 7:56.

8. Albada van S.J., Robinson P.A. Relationships between Electroencephalographic Spectral Peaks Across Frequency Bands. Front Hum Neurosci. 2013 4; 7:56.

9. Andersen P., A. Andersson S. A., Holmgren E. Theoretical consideration on the synchronization of thalamo-cortical activity Subcortical Mechanisms and Sensorimotor Activities / Ed. Frigyesi Bern: Huber. 1975. – P. 229-250.

10. Andrews-Hanna J.R., Smallwood J.N, Spreng R. N. The default network and self-generated thought: component processes, dynamic control, and clinical relevance // Annals of the New York

11. Bailey, S. K.; Aboud, K.S.; Nguyen, T. Q.; C., Laurie E. (13 December 2018). "Applying a network framework to the neurobiology of reading and dyslexia".

Journal of Neurodevelopmental Disorders. 10 (1): 37. doi:10.1186/s11689-018-9251-z. PMC 6291929. PMID 30541433.

12. Bak P, Tang C, Wiesenfeld K. Self-organized criticality: an explanation of the 1/f noise. Phys Rev Lett 1987;27(59):381–4.

13. Barrat A, Barthelemy M, Vespignami A. Dynamical processes on complex networks. Cambridge: Cambridge University Press; 2008

14. Basar E. Brain function and oscillations. – Berlin. New York: Springer. 1998. – 467 p.

15. Basar E., Shurmann M. Alpha rhythms in the brain: functional correlates // News. Physiol. Sci. 1996. V. 11. P. 90–96.

16. Basar E., Shurmann M. Alpha rhythms in the brain: functional correlates // Ns. Physiol. Sci. 1996. V. 11. P. 90–96.

17. Beggs J.M., Plenz D. Neuronal avalanches in neocortical circuits. J Neurosci 2003; 23:11167–77.

18. Bell, Peter T.; Shine, James M. (2015-11-09). "Estimating Large-Scale Network Convergence in the Human Functional Connectome". Brain Connectivity. 5 (9): 565–74. doi:10.1089/brain.2015.0348. PMID 26005099.

19. Bertalanffy Ludwig von The Theory of Open Systems in Physics and Biology// Science 13 January 1950 111: 23-29 [DOI: 10.1126/science.111.2872.23] (in Articles)

20. Besthorn C., Forstl H., Geiger C.-KabischH.SattelT.GasserU.Schreiter-Gasser EEG coherence in Alzheimer disease. Electroencephalography and Clinical Neurophysiology Volume 90, Issue 3, March 1994, Pages 242-245 https://doi.org/10.1016/0013-4694(94)90095-7

21. Boccaletti S, Kurths J, Osipov G, Valladares DL, Zhou CS. The synchronization of chaotic systems. Phys Rep 2002; 366:1–101.

22. Boccaletti S, Kurths J, Osipov G, Valladares DL, Zhou CS. The synchronization of chaotic systems. Phys Rep 2002;366:1–101.

23. Boccaletti S, Latora V, Moreno Y, Chavez M, Hwang D-U. Complex networks: structure and dynamics. Phys Rep 2006;424:175–308.

24. Boccaletti S, Latora V, Moreno Y, Chavez M, Hwang D-U. Complex networks: structure and dynamics. Phys Rep 2006;424:175–308.

25. Bressler, S. L.; Menon, V. (June 2010). "Large scale brain networks in cognition: emerging methods and rprinciples". Trends in Cognitive Sciences. 14 (6): 233–290. doi:10.1016/j.tics.2010.04.004. PMID 20493761. S2CID 5967761. Retrieved 24 January 2016.

26. Bressler, S.L. (2008). "Neurocognitive networks". Scholarpedia. 3 (2): 1567. Bibcode:2008SchpJ...3.1567B. doi:10.4249/scholarpedia.1567.

27. Bressler, Steven L.; Menon, Vinod (June 2010). "Large scale brain networks in cognition: emerging methods and principles". Trends in Cognitive Sciences.14 (6): 233–290. doi:10.1016/j.tics.2010.04.004. PMID 20493761. S2CID 5967761. Retrieved 24 January 2016.

28. Buckner, Randy L. (2012-08-15). "The serendipitous discovery of the brain's default network". NeuroImage. 62 (2): 1137–1145. doi:10.1016/j.neuroimage.2011.10.035. ISSN 1053-119. PMID 22037421. S2CID 9880586.

29. Buckner, R.L., Hanna A., Daniel L. S. The Brain's Default Network Anatomy, Function, and Relevance to Disease. https://doi.org/10.1196/annals.1440.011

30. Bullmore E., Sporns O. The economy of brain network organization- Nature Reviews Neuroscience, 2012 -13 (5): 336-349, http: // dx.doi.org/10.1038/nrn3214.

31. Carracedo L.M., Kjeldsen H., Cunnington L., Jenkins A., Schofield I., Cunningham M.O., Davies C.H., Traub R.D., Whittington M.A. A neocortical delta rhythm facilitates reciprocal interlaminar interactions via nested theta rhythms.J Neurosci. 2013 Jun 26;33(26):10750-61.

32. Cohn R., The occipital alpha rhythm: a study of phase variations / Cohn R. // J.Neurophysiol. – 1948. – V. 11. – P. 31–37.

33. Dubois B. 0[etal m. The 0FAB: am frontal assessmentbatter yatbedside.Neurology, 2000,vol. 55, no. 3, pp. 1621-1626.

34. Eickhoff, S.B.; Yeo, B.T.T., Genon, S., (November 2018). "Imaging-based parcellations of the human brain"(PDF). Nature Reviews. Neuroscience.19 (11): 672–686. doi:10.1038/s41583-018-0071-7.PMID. S2CID 52954265.

35. ElbleR.J. Characteristicof physiologic tremorinyo ungandelderlyadults. J.Clin Neurophysiol, 2003, no.114, suppl. 4, no.624-635.

36. Flor-Henry, P., Koles Z. J. (1982). EEG characteristics of normal subjects: A comparison of men and women and of dextrals and sinistrals. Research Communications in Psychology, Psychiatry & Behavior, 7(1), 21–38.

37. Foster, Brett L.; Parvizi, Josef (2012-03-01). "Resting oscillations and cross-frequency coupling in the human posteromedial cortex". NeuroImage. 60 (1): 384–391. doi:10.1016/j.neuroimage.2011.12.019. ISSN 1053-8119. PMC 3596417. PMID 22227048.

38. Frontiers in Psychology. 3: 295. doi:10.3389/fpsyg.2012.00295. PMC 3427917.PMID 22969735.

39. Gasser T., Christine Jennen-Steinmetz Ch., Rolf Verleger R., EEG coherence at rest and during a visual task in two groups of children Electroencephalography and Clinical Neurophysiology. Volume 67, Issue 2, 1987, P. 151-158.

40. Griffiths, Kristi R.; Braund, Taylor A.; Kohn, Michael R.; Clarke, Simon; Williams, Leanne M.; Korgaonkar, Mayuresh S. (2 March 2021). "Structural brain network topology underpinning ADHD and response to methylphenidate treatment". Translational Psychiatry. 11 (1): 150. doi:10.1038/s41398-021-01278-x. PMC 7925571. PMID 33654073.

41. Growdon W., Ghika J., Henderson J. Effects of proximal and distalmuscles' groups' contraction and mental stress on the amplitude and frequency of physiological finger tremor. Anaccelerometric study. Electromyogr Clin Neurophysiol, 2000, no.40, suppl. 5, pp.295-303.

42. Gurfinkel' V. S., KotsYa. M., Shik M. L. Regulyatsiya pozy cheloveka [Regulation of human posture]. Moscow, Science Publ., 1965, 256 p. (In Russ.)

43. Hallett M. Over view of human tremor physiology. Movement Disorders, 1998, no. 13, suppl. 3, 43-48.

44. Hutton, John S.; Dudley, Jonathan; Horowitz-Kraus, Tzipi; DeWitt, Tom; Holland, Scott K. (1 September 2019)."Functional Connectivity of Attention, Visual, and Language Networks During Audio, Illustrated, and Animated Stories in Preschool-Age Children". Brain Connectivity. 9 (7): 580–592. doi:10.1089/brain.2019.0679. PMC 6775495. PMID 31144523.

45. Buckner R.L., Andrews-Hanna J.R., Schacter D.L. The brain's default network: anatomy, function, and relevance to disease. Annals of the new York Academy of Sciences, 2008•Wiley Online Libra

46. Bassett, Daniella; Bertolero, Max (July 2019). "How Matter Becomes Mind". Scientific American. 321 (1): 32. Retrieved 23 June 2019.

47. Heine, Lizette; Soddu, Andrea; Gomez, Francisco; Vanhaudenhuyse, Audrey; Tshibanda, Luaba; Thonnard, Marie; Charland-Verville, Vanessa; Kirsch, Murielle; Laureys, Steven; Demertzi, Athena (2012)."Resting state networks and consciousness. Alterations of multiple resting state network connectivity in physiological, pharmacological and pathological consciousness sta

48. Kanda P.A.M., Anghinah R., Magali Taino Smidth M.T., Jorge Mario Silva J.M. The clinical use of quantitative EEG in cognitive disorders A utilizacaoclinica do EEG quantitativo nos transtornos cognitivos. Dement. neuropsychol. 3 (3) 2009.
https://doi.org/10.1590/S1980-57642009DN30300004.

49. Khazi M., Kumar A., Dept V.M. Analysis of EEG Using 10:20 Electrode System. International Journal of Innovative Research in Science, Engineering and Technology Vol. 1, Issue 2, 2012.

50. Korenkevych D, Chien J.H., Zhang J. Small world networks in computational neuroscience. Handbook of, 2013 - jhu.pure.elsevier.com

51. Korenkevych D., Chien J.-H, Zhang J., Deng Shan Shiau D,-C,, Chris Sackellares Ch., Pardalos P.M.

52. L. Von Bertalanffy, "General theory of system application to psychology," Soc. Sci. Inform. Sci. Soc., No. 6, 126-136 (1967).

53. Lehmann, D. Human scalp EEG fields:evoked, alpha, sleep and spike-wave patterns / D. Lehmann // Synchronization of EEG Activity in Epilepsies. – New York: Springer-Verlag, 1972. – P. 307-326.

54. Lobasyuk B. A., Bartsevich L. B., Zamkovaya A. V. Application of multiple regression analysis to study the relationship between eeg rhythms at persons with mental retardation. Journal f Education, Health and Sport. 2022;12(2):232-248. Eissn

55. Lobasyuk B.A., Bartsevich L.B., Zamkovaya A.V. Application of multiple regression analysis to study the relationship between eeg rhythms kat persons with mental retardation. Journal of Education, Health and Sport. 2022; 12(2):232-248. eISSN 2391-8306. DOI
http://dx.doi.org/10.12775/JEHS.2022.12.02.025

56. Lobasyuk B.A., Role of the brainstem reticular formation in the mechanisms of cortical electrogenesis. 2005.-Neurophysiology. -V. 37 , №1. – S.39-45.

57. Locatellia T., M.Cursia M., D.Liberatib D.,, M.Franceschia M., Comia G. EEG coherence in Alzheimer's disease Electroencephalography and Clinical Neurophysiology. Volume 106, Issue 3, March 1998, Pages 229-237

58. Lopes da Silva F.H., van Lierop T.H.M.T., Schrijer C.F.M. Storm van Leeuwen W. Essential differences between alpha rhythm and barbiturate spindles: spectra and thalamo-cortical coherence Electroenceph. clin. – 1973b. – V. 35. – P. 626-639.

59. Mangeym B., Rich P.K., Politologiya. Metodyi issledovaniya, Ves Mir, Moskva (1997).

60. Marco-Pallares J., Grau C., Location of brain rhythms and their modulation by preparatory attention estimated by current density C.M.Gomeza Brain Research Volume 1107, Issue 1, 30 August 2006, Pages 151-160.

61. Marek, Scott; Dosenbach, Nico U. F. (June 2018). "The frontoparietal network: function, electrophysiology, and importance of individual precision mapping". Dialogues in Clinical Neuroscience. 20 (2): 133–140.
doi:10.31887/DCNS.2018.20.2/smarek.ISSNm1294-8322.   PMC   6136121. PMID 30250390.

62. McAuleyJ.H., MarsdenC.D. Physiological and pathological tremor sandrhythmic central motor control. Brain, 2000, no. 123, suppl. 8, pp.1545-1567.

63. Menon, V. (2015-01-01), "Salience Network", in Toga, Arthur W. (ed.), Brain Mapping, Academic Press, pp. 597–611, doi:10.1016/B978-0-12-397025-1.00052-X, ISBN 978-0-12-397316-0, retrieved 2019-12-08

64. Menon, Vinod (2011-09-09)."Large-scale brain networks and psychopathology: A unifying triple network model".Trends in Cognitive Sciences. 15 (10): 483–506. doi:10.1016/j.tics.2011.08.003. PMID 21908230. S2CID 26653572.

65. Michael D.; Corbetta, Maurizio; Snyder, Abraham Z.; Vincent, Justin L.; Raichle, Marcus E. (2006-06-27). "Spontaneous neuronal activity distinguishes human dorsal and ventral attention systems". Proceedings of the National Academy of Sciences.103 (26): 10046–10051. Bibcode:2006PNAS..10310046F.doi:10.1073/pnas.0604187103. ISSN 0027-8424. PMC 1480402. PMID 16788060.

66. Michel C.M., Lehmann D., Henggeler B., Brandeis D. Localization of the sources of EEG delta, theta, alpha and beta frequency bands using the FFT dipole approximation.//Electroencephalogr Clin Neurophysiol. 1992; 82(1):38-44.

67. Michel C.M., Lehmann D., Henggeler B., Brandeis D. Localization of the sources of EEG delta, theta, alpha and beta frequency bands using the FFT dipole approximation.//Electroencephalogr Clin Neurophysiol. 1992; 82(1):38-44.

68. Morris, Peter G.; Smith, Stephen M.; Barnes, Gareth R.; Stephenson, Mary C.; Hale, Joanne R.; Price, Darren; Luckhoo, Henry; Woolrich, Mark; Brookes, Matthew J. (2011-10-04)."Investigating the electrophysiological basis of resting state networks using magnetoencephalography". Proceedings of the National Academy of Sciences. 108 (40): 16783–16788. Bibcode:2011PNAS.10816783B.doi:10.1073/pnas.1112685108. ISSN 0027-8424.PMC 3189080. PMID 21930901.

69. n S.A. Thalamic origin of cortical rhythmic activity / Handbook of Electroencephalography and Clinical Neurophysiology / Ed. Amsterdam: Elsevier. 1974. – Vol. 2, – P. 90

70. Network". Annals of the New York Academy of Sciences. 1124 (1): 1–38. Bibcode:2008NYASA1124....1B. doi:10.1196/annals.1440.011. ISSN 1749-6632. PMID 18400922. S2CID 3167595.

71. Nunez PL. Brain, mind, and the structure of reality. Oxford University Press; 2010.

72. O'Suilleabhain P.E., Matsumoto J.Y. Time-frequency analysis of tremors. Brain, 1998, no. 121, pp. 2127-2124.

73. Pardalos V: Du P.M, Graham D.-Z., RL (editors). Combinatorial Optimization Reference. New York: Springer; 2013; p. 3057-3088

74. Petersen, Steven; Sporns, Olaf (October 2015)."Brain Networks and Cognitive Architectures". Neuron. 88 (1): 207–219. doi:10.1016/j.neuron.2015.09.027. PMC 4598639. PMID 26447582.

75. Petersen, Steven; Sporns, Olaf (October 2015). "Brain Networks and Cognitive Architectures". Neuron. 88 (1): 207–219. doi:10.1016/j.neuron.2015.09.027. PMC 4598639. PMID 26447582.

76. Raethjen J., Pawlas F., Lindemann M. [et al.] Determinants of physiologic tremor in a large normal population. J.ClinNeurophysiol, 2000, no. 111, suppl. 10, pp. 1825-1837

77. Raichle Marcus E. The Brain's Default Mode Network // Annual Review of Neuroscience. — 2015.— Vol. 38. — P. 433-447. — ISSN 0147-006X. — doi:10.1146/annurev-neuro-071013-014030

78. Raichle Marcus E. The Brain's Default Mode Network // Annual Review of Neuroscience. — 2015. — Vol.38. — P.433-447.—ISSN 0147-006X.— doi:10.1146/annurev-neuro-071013-014030

79. Riedl V.; Utz L.; Castrillon G. et sll. 2016; Bressler Steven L.; Menon, V. 2010; Yeo, B. T. Thomas; Krienen, Fenna M.; Sepulcre J. 2011).

80. Riedl V., Utz L. C., Gabriel G., Timo R, J. P.; Ploner M.F., Friston, K.J.; Drzezga A., Sorg Ch. (January 12, 2016)."Metabolic connectivity mapping reveals effective connectivity in the resting human brain". PNAS. 113(2): 428–433.Bibcode:2016PNAS..113..428R. doi:10.1073/pnas.1513752113. PMC 4720331. PMID 26712010.

81. Riedl, Valentin; Utz, Lukas; Castrillon, Gabriel; Grimmer, Timo; Rauschecker, Josef P.; Ploner, Markus; Friston, Karl J.; Drzezga, Alexander; Sorg, Christian (January 12, 2016). "Metabolic connectivity mapping reveals effective connectivity in the resting human brain". PNAS. 113 (2): 428–433. Bibcode:2016PNAS, 113. 428R. doi:10.1073/pnas.1513752113. PMC 4720331. PMID 26712010.

82. Riedl, Valentin; Utz, Lukas; Castrillon, Gabriel; Grimmer, Timo; Rauschecker, Josef P.; Ploner, Markus; Friston, Karl J.; Drzezga, Alexander; Sorg, Christian (January 12, 2016). "Metabolic connectivity mapping reveals effective connectivity in the resting human brain". PNAS. 113 (2): 428–433. Bibcode:2016PNAS, 113. 428R. doi:10.1073/pnas.1513752113. PMC 4720331. PMID 26712010.

83. S. J. Williamson, L. Kaufman, Z.-L. Lu, et al., "Study of human occipital alpha rhythm: the alphon hypothesis and alpha suppression," Int. J. Psychophysiol., 26(1-3), 63-76 (1997).

84. S.A. Isaychev, D.S. Osipova , Yu.M. Koptelov. Dipolnyie modeli generatora alfa-ritma. Fiziol. Vyissh. Nervnoy (psihicheskoy) deyatelnosti. 2003. T.53. #5. s. 577-586.

85. Scolari, Miranda; Seidl-Rathkopf, Katharina N; Kastner, Sabine (2015-02-01). "Functions of the human frontoparietal attention network: Evidence from neuroimaging". Current Opinion in Behavioral Sciences. Cognitive control. 1: 32–39. doi:10.1016/j.cobeha.2014.08.003. ISSN 2352-1546. PMC 4936532. PMID 27398396.

86. Shafiei, Golia; Zeighami, Yashar; Clark, Crystal A.; Coull, Jennifer T.; Nagano-Saito, Atsuko; Leyton, Marco; Dagher, Alain; Misic, Bratislav (2018-10-01). "Dopamine Signaling Modulates the Stability and Integration of Intrinsic Brain Networks". Cerebral Cortex. 29 (1): 397–409. doi:10.1093/cercor/bhy264. PMC 6294404. PMID 30357316.

87. Shannon CE, Weaver W. The mathematical theory of communication. Urbana and Chicago: University of Illinois Press; 1949.

88. Shaw J.C., O'Connor K.P., Ongley C. The EEG as a measure of cerebral functional organization.- The British Journal of Psychiatry, 1977 – 130 (3): 260-264)

89. Shulman, Gordon L.; McAvoy, Mark P.; Cowan, Melanie C.; Astafiev, Serguei V.; Tansy, Aaron P.; d'Avossa, Giovanni; Corbetta, Maurizio (2003-11-01). "Quantitative Analysis of Attention and Detection Signals During Visual Search". Journal of Neurophysiology. 90 (5): 3384–3397. doi:10.1152/jn.00343.2003. ISSN 0022-3077. PMID 12917383.

90. Simon HA. The architecture of complexity. Proc Natl Acad Sci USA 1962; 106:467–82. Simpson Small world networks in computational neuroscience

91. 91.   Small world networks in computational neuroscience V: Pardalos P.M, Du D.-Z., Graham RL (editors). Combinatorial Optimization Reference. New York: Springer; 2013; p. 3057-3088

92. Smith, S.M.; Fox, P.T.; Miller, K.L. et al) .10-15). "Evaluation of the spatial variability in the major resting-state networks across human brain functional atlases". Human Brain Mapping. 40 (15): 4577–4587. doi:10.1002/hbm.24722. PMC 6771873. PMID 31322303.

93. Smith, SM; Fox, PT; Miller, KL; Glahn, DC; Fox, PM; Mackay, CE; Filippini, N; Watkins, KE; Toro, R; Laird, AR; Beckmann, CF (2009-08-04). "Correspondence of the brain's functional architecture during activation and rest". Proceedings of the National Academy of Sciences of the United States of America. 106 (31): 13040–5. Bibcode:2009PNAS.10613040S. doi:10.1073/pnas.0905267106. PMC 2722273. PMID 19620724.

94. Smith, SM; Fox, PT; Miller, KL; Glahn, DC; Fox, PM; Mackay, CE; Filippini, N; Watkins, KE; Toro, R; Laird, AR; Beckmann, CF (2009-08-04). "Correspondence of the brain's functional architecture during activation and rest". Proceedings of the National Academy of Sciences of the United States of America. 106 (31): 13040–Bibcode:2009PNAS..10613040S. doi:10.1073/pnas.0905267106. PMC 2722273. PMID 19620724.

95. Sporns O, Tononi G, Edelman GM. Theoretical neuroanatomy: relating anatomical and functional connectivity in graphs and cortical connection matrices. Cereb Cortex 2000; 10:127–41. Sporns O, Kotter R. Motifs in brain networks. PLoS Biol 2004; 2:e369.

96. Sporns O. Complex network measures of brain connectivity: uses and interpretations. Neuroimage 2010; 52:1059–69.

97. Sporns O. Networks of the brain. Cambridge, Massachusetts: The MIT Press; 2011a.

98. Sporns O. The human connectome: a complex network. Ann NY Acad Sci 2011b; 1224:109–25.

99. Stam CJ. Nonlinear dynamical analysis of EEG and MEG: review of an emerging field. Clin Neurophysiol 2005; 116:2266–301.

100. Stam, E.C.W. van Straaten / Clinical Neurophysiology xxx (2012) xxx–xxx Please cite this article in press as: Stam CJ, van Straaten ECW. The organization of physiological brain networks. Clin Neurophysiol (2012), doi:10.1016/j.clinph.2012.01.011

101. Steimke, Rosa; Nomi, Jason S.; Calhoun, Vince D.; Stelzel, Christine; Paschke, Lena M.; Gaschler, Robert; Goschke, Thomas; Walter, Henrik; Uddin, Lucina Q. (2017-12-01). "Salience network dynamics underlying successful resistance of temptation". Social Cognitive and Affective Neuroscience. 12 (12): 1928–1939. doi:10.1093/scan/nsx123. ISSN 1749-5016. PMC 5716209. PMID 29048582.

102. Thomas B. T; Krienen, Fenna M.; Sepulcre, Jorge; Sabuncu, Mert R.; Lashkari Danial; Hollinshead, Marisa; Roffman, Joshua L.; Smoller, Jordan W.; Zollei, Lilla; Polimeni, Jonathan R.; Fischl, Bruce; Liu, Hesheng; Buckner, Randy L. (2011, -09-01). "The organization of the human cerebral cortex estimated by intrinsic functional connectivity". Journal of Neurophysiology. 106 (3): 1125–1165. Bibcode:2011NatSD...2E0031H. doi:10.1152/jn.00338.2011. PMC 3174820. PMID 21653723.

103. Tucker M., Stenslie C.E., Randy S. Roth R.S., MS; Steve L. Shearer S.l. Right Frontal Lobe Activation and Right Hemisphere PerformanceDecrement During

a Depressed Mood Arch Gen Psychiatry. 1981;38(2):169-174. doi:10.1001/archpsyc.1981.01780270055007

104. Uddin, L.Q.; Yes, BTT; Spreng, R.N. (November 2019). "Towards a universal taxonomy of macroscale functional networks in the human brain". Topography of the brain. 32(6): 926–942. doi:10.1007/s10548-019-6. PMC 7325607. PMID31707621

105. Uddin, LQ; Yeo, BTT; Spreng, RN (November 2019). "Towards a Universal Taxonomy of Macro-scale Functional Human Brain Networks". Brain Topography. 32 (6): 926–942. doi:10.1007/s10548-019-00744-6. PMC 7325607. PMID 31707621.

106. Uddin, LQ; Yeo, BTT; Spreng, RN (November 2019). "Towards a Universal Taxonomy of Macro-scale Functional Human Brain Networks". Brain Topography. 32 (6): 926–942. doi:10.1007/s10548-019-00744-6. PMC 7325607. PMID 31707621.

107. Uddin, Lucina (10 October 2022). "The Brain Network by Any Other Name". Journal of Cognitive Neuroscience. 2022 (10): 363–364. doi: 10.1162/jocn_a_01925. PMID 36223250. S2CID 252844955

108. Uddin, Lucina (2022-10-10). "A Brain Network by Any Other Name". Journal of Cognitive Neuroscience. 2022 (10): 363–364. doi:10.1162/jocn_a_01925. PMID 36223250. S2CID 25284495

109. Uddin, Lucina (2022-10-10). "A Brain Network by Any Other Name". Journal of Cognitive Neuroscience. 2022 (10): 363–364. doi:10.1162/jocn_a_01925. PMID 36223250. S2CID 252844955.

110. von Bertalanffy L. General system theory. Foundations, development, applications. New York: George Braziller

111. Vossel, Simone; Geng, Joy J.; Fink, Gereon R. (2014). "Dorsal and Ventral Attention Systems: Distinct Neural Circuits but Collaborative Roles". The Neuroscientist. 20 (2): 150–159. doi:10.1177/1073858413494269. PMC 4107817. PMID 23835449.

112. Weiss S., Rappelsberger P. Left Frontal EEG Coherence Reflects Modality Independent Language Processes // Brain Topograpy. 1998. Vol. 11. № 1. P. 33–42

113. Weiss S., Rappelsberger P. Left Frontal EEG Coherence Reflects Modality Independent Language Processes // Brain Topograpy. 1998. Vol. 11. № 1. P. 33–42

114. Weiss S., Rappelsberger P. Left Frontal EEG Coherence Reflects Modality Independent Language Processes // Brain Topograpy 1998. Vol. 11. № 1. P. 33–42ith

115. Wiener N. Cybernetics: or control and communication in the animal and the machine. Cambridge, Massachusetts: The MIT Press; 1948.

116. Williamson S. J., Kaufman L., Lu Z.-L., et al., tudy of human occipital alpha rhythm: the alphon hypothesis and alpha suppression,Int. J. Psychophysiol., 26(1-3), 63-76 (1997)

117. Yang, Yan-li; Deng, Hong-xia; Xing, Gui-yang; Xia, Xiao-luan; Li, Hai-fang (2015). "Brain functional network connectivity based on a visual task: visual information processing-related brain regions are significantly activated in the task state". Neural Regeneration Research. 10 (2): 298–307. doi:10.4103/1673-5374.152386. PMC 4392680. PMID 25883631.

118. Yeo, B. T. Thomas; Krienen, Fenna M.; Sepulcre, Jorge; Sabuncu, Mert R.; Lashkari, Danial; Hollinshead, Marisa; Roffman, Joshua L.; Smoller, ordan W.; Zollei, Lilla; Polimeni, Jonathan R.; Fischl, Bruce; Liu, Hesheng; Buckner, Randy L. (2011-09-01). "The organization of the human cerebral cortex estimated by intrinsic functional connectivity". Journal of Neurophysiology. 106 (3): 1125–1165. Bibcode:2011NatSD...2E0031H. doi:10.1152/jn.00338.2011. PMC 3174820. PMID 21653723.

119. Yuan, Rui; Di, Xin; Taylor, Paul A.; Gohel, Suril; Tsai, Yuan-Hsiung; Biswal, Bharat B. (30 April 2015). "Functional topography of the thalamocortical system in human". Brain Structure and Function. 221 (4): 1971–1984. doi:10.1007/s00429-015-1018-7. PMC 6363530. PMID 25924563.

120. Zheng-yan Jiang Study on EEG power and coherence in patients with mild cognitive impairment during working memory task. Journal of Zhejiang University SCIENCE